Unjunk Your Junk Food

Unjunk Your Junk Food

HEALTHY ALTERNATIVES TO CONVENTIONAL SNACKS

Andrea Donsky and Randy Boyer
with Lisa Tsakos

Gallery Books 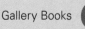 New York London Toronto Sydney New Delhi

G

Gallery Books

A Division of Simon & Schuster, Inc.

1230 Avenue of the Americas

New York, NY 10020

First Gallery Books trade paperback edition January 2012

GALLERY BOOKS and colophon are registered trademarks of Simon & Schuster, Inc.

For information about special discounts for bulk purchases, please contact Simon & Schuster Special Sales at 1-866-506-1949 or business@simonandschuster.com.

The Simon & Schuster Speakers Bureau can bring authors to your live event. For more information or to book an event, contact the Simon & Schuster Speakers Bureau at 1-866-248-3049 or visit our website at www.simonspeakers.com.

Manufactured in the United States of America

10 9 8 7 6 5 4 3 2 1

Library of Congress Cataloging-in-Publication Data

Donsky, Andrea.
    Unjunk your junk food : healthy alternatives to conventional snacks /
Andrea Donsky and Randy Boyer ; with Lisa Tsakos. — 1st Gallery Books trade pbk. ed.
        p.   cm.
    Includes bibliographical references and index.
    1. Snack foods.   2. Natural foods.   I. Boyer, Randy.   II. Tsakos, Lisa.   III. Title.
TX740.D645   2011
642—dc23   2011026277

ISBN 978-1-4516-1656-9
ISBN 978-1-4516-1660-6 (ebook)

A Note to the Reader

Acknowledgments

Who would have thought that our mutual love for junk food and natural health would have turned into a book? We're so happy that life's twists and turns brought us to this very moment, but we didn't get here alone. There are many people we'd like to thank for helping us with this book:

Our Publisher, Simon & Schuster

Thank you for believing in our concept, getting excited about the idea and about NaturallySavvy.com, and your passion for educating readers. Special thanks to: Jen Bergstrom, Kathy Sagan, Jamie Putorti, Nancy Inglis, and Natasha Simons.

Our Literary Agents

Kristina Holmes and Michael Ebeling: You believed in us, had the foresight to suggest a book, offered wonderful feedback, put in a lot of hard work, and were oh-so-patient with us for two years. Thank you for your endless encouragement.

Dr. David Katz: Thank you for introducing us to Kristina and Michael well before we even knew what type of book we wanted to write.

Our Research Team

Kristen Mehendale, Avery Pawelek, Elana Davis, Erin Moore, Kimie Ando, Dan Ransom, Natalie Maurice, Nahid Ameen, Tamara Junkin, Lindsay Tadros: You all have our sincere thanks for countless hours of organization, feedback, patience, and of course, fact finding—the very foundations of this book.

Our Support Team

Bruce Bechtel, Jim Empey, Lorene Sauro, Chuck Cassidy, Rhonda Lewis, Dawn at NaturalCandyStore.com: Thank you for being there when we had questions we couldn't answer on our own or facts we needed to check on.

Our Taste Testers

Lisa Goldenberg, Maureen Taran, Erika Hurwitz: It's a tough job, but somebody had to do it! Your willingness to try anything was astounding, and your honest feedback was (and is) ever so much appreciated.

Our Editorial Team

Cara Smusiak, Sara Vigneri, Matt Hartley: Detailed, thorough, and willing to work into the wee hours, on weekends, and at the drop of a hat—could we ask for more? Your work made this book sparkle like a diamond, and for that we give you our heartfelt thanks.

Our Artistic Talent

Lisa Simonsen: Thank you for bringing our concept to life with a beautifully designed proposal and cover—we might not have had a book without it!

Tirzah Tward: Our brilliant designer, who worked endlessly for weeks to create our beautiful book. We appreciate you.

Jessica Heald: Thank you for helping us meet our design deadline.

Our Stylist and Photographers

Rinat Samuel: We're forever in your debt for making us look so savvy and stunning for our photo shoot.

Alison Vieira: We truly appreciate your amazing talent with the camera. Your photos of us are wonderful.

Joanne Tsakos: You handled the never-ending product photo shoots gracefully. Thank you for making the products look so captivating.

Our Savvy Chef

Claire Fountain: Thank you for whipping up healthy and delicious recipes our readers will love!

Our Families

To our wonderful husbands: While we know each of you wants the top acknowledgment, you are all amazing and understanding. Never complaining about our late nights, entertaining the kiddies after hours, giving your honest feedback about the products (Howard and Rich: you were the best at that), and even taking the little ones on weeklong trips (we're looking at you, Jason), we love and appreciate the three of you.

To our kids: We could always count on you to help us with sampling and feedback of all the products we received (like we could have stopped you!), put up with our absence, and happily take care of Olivia and baby Abby while we were working. We love you, forever and always.

Introduction: Getting Your Fix

Chances are if you're reading this book, you've got something of a sweet (or salty?) tooth. That's all right—we do too! Whether it's curling up with a big bowl of buttered popcorn on movie night, taking the kids out for ice cream, or indulging in a gooey chocolate chip cookie straight from the oven, we can't help it. Even the healthiest of health nuts need their junk food fix every now and again.

We're not going to tell you that it's wrong to eat ice cream, that French fries are bad for you, or that you need to ban all cookies from your diet. That's not what this book is about. Let's face it, we love junk food, and we're not afraid to admit it. We assume you're aware of the general health risks that can come along with eating a lot of processed snacks—the dangers of a diet high in sugar, fat, and sodium—so we won't bore you with a lecture. Instead we're here to tell you there are many yummy alternatives available, made with much better quality ingredients. You *can* have your cake and eat it too. Think of this book as a way of getting your junk food fix without all the unhealthy stuff.

When people find out we eat natural and organic products, they usually comment on how disciplined we must be for opting to eat such tasteless, boring, and highly restrictive foods. This couldn't be further from the truth. Having embraced such foods for over a decade, we know how tasty and satisfying they can be. Our own kitchens are stocked with a wide array of snacks that aren't much different from those in any other homes. Our kids love cookies, our husbands munch on chips, we love candy and chocolate, and we often serve cake for dessert. The only difference is the brands we choose. Instead of Kellogg's Pop-Tarts, Nabisco Oreos, and Nestlé Drumstick ice-cream sundae cones, we buy Nature's Path Organic Toaster Pastries, Country Choice Organic Sandwich Cremes chocolate cookies, and Turtle Mountain Purely Decadent Coconut Milk Non-Dairy Frozen Dessert. Make no mistake: the healthier brands we choose taste great, too!

To write this book, the Naturally Savvy team rigorously taste tested each product in the guide. (We admit: it was a tough job sampling all that junk food.) Together we ranked and reviewed hundreds of conventional, natural, and organic snack foods, comparing the quality of their ingredients and flavor in search of the healthiest alternatives for the treats we love.

Our chief nutrition expert, Lisa Tsakos, carefully examined every label to identify unhealthy ingredients such as partially hydrogenated oils (trans fats) and artificial sweeteners, colorings, and flavors. (See chapter 3, "The Worst Ingredients.") Products that met our guidelines received the Naturally Savvy Seal of Approval™.

Our Seal of Approval helps identify the healthier options, while omitting their unhealthy alternatives, thereby eliminating the guesswork for you.

We wrote *Unjunk Your Junk Food* for the same reason we created our website, NaturallySavvy.com: to tell you that you don't have to give up what you love best. You just have to make smart choices. Our goal is to empower you with the tools you need to make healthy food choices. As the poet Dr. Maya Angelou said, "When you know better, you do better."

The truth is, there are no shortcuts to healthy eating. But it really is easier than you may think. Once you understand the basics of good nutrition, you'll know how to interpret what's listed on a food label and how to focus on what's important.

The key is to know *how* to decipher the nutrition label. Instead of immediately looking at the *quantity* (calories, fat, and serving size), look first at the *quality* of the ingredients (nutrients, chemical preservatives, artificial additives, and food colorings). Although junk food can evoke warm and fuzzy feelings, many of our favorite snack foods are filled with artificial, unhealthy, and sometimes dangerous ingredients.

The good news is now there are healthier junk food options made without chemical preservatives, food colorings, artificial flavors, high-fructose corn syrup, and trans fats. And the best part is that you don't sacrifice on taste. Of course, eating healthier junk food isn't a license to eat as much of it as you want; as always, moderation is key. Happy munching and crunching!

In good health,

Andrea Donsky & Randy Boyer
Co-founders, NaturallySavvy.com

Visit www.naturallysavvy.com often for up-to-date articles, blogs, videos, product reviews, and free gifts. For the latest Naturally Savvy updates, sign up for our weekly newsletter, follow us on Twitter (http://twitter.com/ NaturallySavvy), and become a fan on Facebook (www.facebook.com/ NaturallySavvy). Join our forum. Talk to our experts. Ask questions. Have fun.

A Note from the Authors: How to Read This Book

This book is intended as a user-friendly reference guide when planning your grocery shopping and to take with you to the supermarket. When shopping for snacks, flip to the chapter associated with the snack you wish to purchase (potato chips or ice cream, for example), and take a moment to review the ingredients you should watch out for. Many of the "clean" products—meaning those without chemical additives (artificial colors, preservatives, etc.)—are now found in the aisles next to the more popular products, but some supermarkets designate separate areas for natural foods and products.

Each chapter is divided by category. Products are compared side by side: the brand listed on the left page contains unhealthy ingredients, while the brand on the right page lists the better, cleaner option. Our goal is to encourage you to first read the ingredients before looking at the Nutrition Facts panel (or anything else on the package).

❖ **Bad Choice Seal:** This product contains questionable ingredients that we recommend avoiding.

❖ **Ingredients:** The ingredients written in red represent the worst (most dangerous) ingredients. Those in yellow represent questionable ingredients that we recommend avoiding whenever possible.

❖ **Thumbs-down:** This symbol signifies a negative point that we want to call attention to.

❖ **Thumbs-up:** This indicates a positive quality or change.

✥ **Thumbs neutral:** This represents a fact about the conventional product or an ingredient it contains. There is no negative or positive point associated with it.

✥ **Naturally Savvy Seal of Approval™:** Products that met our guidelines received this seal, which helps identify the healthier options while omitting their unhealthy alternatives, thereby eliminating the guesswork for you.

✥ **Savvy Pick:** This explains why we selected a product as the better option. What was most important to us was that our recommended Savvy Picks had no red flag in their ingredients. Several of the natural brands contain yellow flags, but we still felt they were the best option of the natural brands that matched the popular brand.

✥ **Honorable Mention:** A list of runners-up of brands that we approve and that you should also consider trying.

Many large food manufacturers have already begun removing the "bad" ingredients from their products. This is primarily due to consumer complaints. We encourage you to keep asking companies to make cleaner products. We believe they are listening.

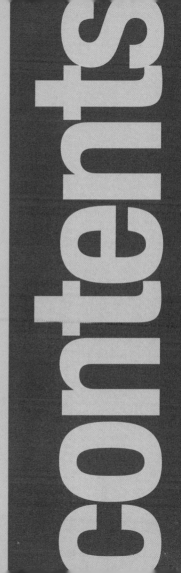
contents

Unjunk Your
Junk Food

the key to unjunking

Statistics show that junk food makes up almost one-third of our daily diet, but while we like our junk, it doesn't really like us. The fallout? Obesity rates are skyrocketing, type 2 diabetes is on the rise, unprecedented numbers of kids are suffering from digestive problems, and global cancer rates are increasing. The thing is, it doesn't have to be this way. We can get back to the basics—back to a cleaner, more nutritious diet that provides a foundation for good health—and still enjoy our snacks.

The key is to choose foods that are minimally processed or prepared without unnecessary chemicals and additives, and to eliminate artificial ingredients as much as you possibly can. The food industry promotes these as "natural foods," but these days you have to be alert even when you see that term. Once used exclusively to describe whole fruits and vegetables and unrefined grains, manufacturers now use the word *natural* for processed foods, many of which can contain a wide array of chemicals.

Using extra ingredients to enhance food is not new. Our ancestors used salts to preserve meat and sugar to preserve fruit. Spices and herbs were used for flavoring, and vegetables were fermented or pickled so that they could be eaten during colder seasons; but the growth of food science as an industry has exploded the amount of processed foods in general—and chemical additives in particular—available in the marketplace. Some synthetic chemicals are harmless. However, others have unknown or even harmful side effects.

Although additives are regulated by federal authorities to ensure that foods are labeled accurately, not all additives have been adequately tested for long-term safety. Consumers have been linking health and behavioral issues to various food additives for decades; unfortunately, their complaints have largely been dismissed by government and the food industry. So ultimately it's up to you to check what ingredients are in the food you are snacking on, especially if it comes in a box or a can. The first step in screening your junk food is to understand exactly what food labels and nutrition panels mean, and use them to help make healthy choices.

Do You Recognize Each Ingredient on a Food Label?

In a recent survey, 55 percent of consumers admitted that they don't understand the meaning of half the ingredients in foods these days! Is that really any surprise? Hundreds of synthetic additives, preservatives, and colorings—with names that we don't recognize—are used to process our food to make it taste better, look more appealing, and last longer.

Before looking at the calories, fat, or anything else on the Nutrition Facts panel, read the ingredients list. Look for any partially hydrogenated oil (the source of trans fat), food coloring (artificial colors), monosodium glutamate (MSG), and artificial sweeteners. If any of these offenders are listed, our advice is to put the snack back on the shelf. If you need more convincing, read chapter 3, "The Worst Ingredients."

Making Sense of Food Labels

Ingredients First

When shopping for groceries—and that includes junk food—check out a product's ingredients list before buying it.

The law requires that a food's ingredients be listed on its label. Ingredients appear in descending order by weight: the one that weighs the most is listed first, the one that weighs the least is last, and so on. Ingredients that make up less than 2 percent of the food by weight are also listed at the end. These may include flavor enhancers, stabilizers, and other chemical agents. Just because they are listed at the end, however, doesn't make them any less dangerous.

Nutrition Next

Once you're satisfied that the ingredients are healthy enough, then look for the following on the package:

1. Calories: Junk food, by its nature, is filled with sugar and/or other empty calories, providing little or no nutritional value. If calories are your big focus, be mindful of the serving size. Most of your daily calorie intake should come from whole foods. (Follow the 80–20 rule: 80 percent quality, 20 percent indulgence.) Sometimes just a taste can be as satisfying as eating the whole thing, but denying yourself completely can lead to binge eating for some people—which isn't remotely healthy.

2. Fat: The type of fat is more important than the amount. The term "partially hydrogenated" is just another way to say "trans fat," the unhealthiest type of fat. This unnatural form of fat has been proven to lead to heart disease, colon cancer, and diabetes.

3. Sodium: Natural or not, sodium is found in most packaged foods. Sodium can cause water retention and affect blood pressure, raising your risk of stroke. Our recommendation is to limit your daily intake to 1,500 milligrams (mg) from all sources, which is far less than the FDA's current recommended maximum of 2,400 milligrams. You can easily exceed both our and the FDA's recommended limits without ever using a saltshaker if you don't keep track of the sodium in the processed foods you eat.

4. Fiber: Fiber is the undigestible portion of carbohydrates. Found naturally in plant foods (vegetables, fruit, beans, nuts, seeds, and whole grains), fiber is a key nutrient in a daily diet. Eating fiber-rich foods not only helps to regulate your digestive system and blood sugar levels (refer to page 10 for an explanation) but also is a low-calorie way to fill your tummy. The average diet provides only about 12 grams of fiber each day, but female adults should consume 35 grams, and males, 38 grams. The higher the amount you find in a single food, the better! So if you come across junk food with 3 or more grams per serving, you've hit the fiber jackpot.

5. Sugar: Junk food is synonymous with sugar, and since we're all aware of the health implications of sugar, here are some simple rules about the sweet stuff: avoid high-fructose corn syrup; always combine sugar (or any form of carbohydrate) with some protein (or a lot of fiber) to prevent spikes in your blood sugar, and look for hidden sources of sugar on food labels. Cane juice, fruit juice concentrate, and corn syrup are just a few of the many forms of sugar found in food products.

Know Your Label Terms

Enriched: This means that a food has had certain nutrients removed, then re-added. An example is adding bran back into refined flour products to increase the fiber content. The question we really need to ask is: "Why did they take it out in the first place?" Typically, it's to prolong the shelf life of a food.

Fat-free: The product contains less than 0.5 grams of fat per serving.

Fortified: When a nutrient has been added to a food that doesn't contain it naturally, the food is said to be fortified. Most of us could use the additional nutrients, but this is done mainly to prevent deficiency diseases such as pellagra or beriberi in those who eat a diet with poor nutritional value.

No Label?
Be leery of packaging with no ingredients listed; for example, sample packs or loot bag treats. A legal loophole exempts small packages from listing their ingredients. Our rule of thumb is, if you don't know what's inside a package, don't eat it.

Knowing the meaning of the words that manufacturers use on food labels empowers you to understand exactly what you are eating. Here are the most frequently used terms you'll come across:

Lite or light: This means that the product contains one-third of the calories or half (or less) the fat of the full-fat version; or half the sodium (or less) of the full-salt version if it states "Lite in sodium." Compare the "light/lite" product with the regular product to see the difference. Sometimes chemicals such as olestra, an artificial fat substitute, are added to reduce the calories of the product. You have to decide if possible side effects of the additive—which can include abdominal cramping and loose stools—offset the benefit of reduced calories.

Low cholesterol: The product contains 20 milligrams or less of cholesterol, and 2 grams or less of saturated fat (see page 9 for a description) per serving. However, it does *not* mean that the product is low in fat, although it must not contain more than 13 grams of fat.

Low-fat: The product contains no more than 3 grams of fat per serving.

Made with organic ingredients: This label guarantees that at least 70 percent of a product's ingredients are organic (refer to the term "organic" in this section for a definition). Products containing less than 70 percent organic ingredients cannot make any claims on the front label but may list the organic ingredients on the back panel.

No added sugar: This sounds good, but the product may already contain sugar *naturally*.

No salt added: While no *salt* has been added, it doesn't mean that other sodium sources have not been added, or that a product isn't naturally high in sodium.

Organic: This word tells you that the food or product is guaranteed to contain at least 95 percent organic ingredients measured by weight. Any nonorganic ingredients, up to a maximum of 5 percent, must still receive approval from the US Department of Agriculture's National Organic Program (NOP), which develops and administers national labeling standards. These products may display the USDA Organic seal. For the USDA's definition of organic and to learn more about the National Organic Program, visit their website: www.ams.usda.gov/nop.

100 percent organic: This means that a product is made with 100 percent organic ingredients. This is the highest standard of organic, and you can rest assured that these products are, in fact, completely organic.

Reduced or less fat: The product has at least 25 percent less fat than the full-fat product.

Salt free: Check the Nutrition Facts panel to determine the amount of sodium per serving, and look for sodium sources other than salt, such as MSG.

Sugar free: This means that a food can contain up to 0.5 grams of sugar per serving. Second, it can contain artificial sweeteners such as aspartame, sucralose (Splenda), and others that are also not great for you.

Visit the USDA's website at www.fda.gov for more details about food labels.

How Trustworthy Is the Nutrition Panel?

To verify the nutrition facts and ingredients, we contacted every company individually. Interestingly, a few of the major food manufacturers weren't forthcoming with their ingredients. We were surprised by the poor level of customer service we often encountered. Many calls were disconnected or weren't returned. Customer service employees weren't aware of (or couldn't pronounce) several of the ingredients in their own products, or had no idea where to find updated ingredients lists.

This concerned us and sparked many conversations about how challenging it might be for someone with severe allergies to obtain accurate ingredient information that could prevent a reaction. To be extra diligent, we took all the information directly from the packages, so if there are any discrepancies, it's because companies may have reformulated their ingredients after we bought the products.

back-to-basics nutrition

2

*T*o stay healthy you need to eat a diet that includes the right amount of carbohydrates, protein, fats, fiber, and vitamins and minerals. Here's the rundown:

The Well-Balanced Diet

1. Carbohydrates—The Fuel: Carbohydrates such as fruits, vegetables, whole grains, beans, and lentils are the body's primary source of energy. Despite what some weight loss programs suggest, you need carbs. But if you eat too many, or you eat the wrong type, the body produces extra insulin, the hormone that travels through the bloodstream delivering glucose to all the body's cells. This drives down your blood sugar levels, leading to a vicious cycle:

Eat too many carbs (sugar) → which results in high blood sugar levels → which leads to an overproduction of insulin → which works to lower blood sugar levels → and we end up craving sweets and other carbs in order to bring our blood sugar levels back to normal.

This unhealthy cycle will eventually lead to weight gain and insulin resistance—the body's reduced ability to respond to the effects of insulin. As a result, the body needs more insulin to help glucose enter cells, causing a buildup of glucose in the bloodstream and setting the stage for type 2 diabetes. Long before that happens, however, the effects of sugar take their toll. Sugar increases the "bad" intestinal bacteria that suppress the immune system and make us more susceptible to infections and illness. All carbohydrates, no matter the source, are ultimately broken down into glucose (sugar), which is either burned for energy immediately or stored in the liver, the muscles, and our fat cells for long-term storage. So if you eat too many high-carb foods, the body stores them as fat—unless, of course, you exercise avidly. It's that simple.

Glycemic Index (GI): Low Is the Way to Go

Not all carbs are created equal. "Simple carbs" from refined and processed foods (think "white" foods such as white bread and white rice), junk food, and sweets are quickly absorbed by the blood, whereas sugars from complex carbohydrates—vegetables, whole grains, legumes, and fruits enter the bloodstream more slowly. The glycemic index (GI) can help you choose the right carbs to eat.

The GI measures the effect of a given carbohydrate on your blood sugar on a scale from 0 to 100. Foods with a high GI result in noticeable fluctuations in blood sugar levels, which raise insulin levels. Low GI foods are slower to digest and raise blood sugar levels more slowly. You can't go wrong if you concentrate on foods with lower GI scores.

To take it one step further, the *glycemic load* measures the quantity of carbs in the measured portion of food as compared to the GI. There are many resources available on the Internet and at bookstores and libraries to help you understand the glycemic index and the glycemic load.

2. Protein—The Power Source: How much protein do you need? There is tremendous variation in daily protein requirements. Protein should account for 10 percent to 35 percent of your daily caloric intake. To determine whether your needs should be closer to the high or the low, consider your activity level, lean body (muscle) mass, the type of protein you eat, your age, and your health status.

Dietary protein is not stored as fat like sugars, carbs, and fats are. Building dinners around protein and plenty of vegetables is a healthy and fast approach to weight loss.

Having a protein-rich breakfast within thirty minutes of waking up will help get your brain working. It will also help stabilize your blood sugar, preventing blood-sugar-related mood swings and energy dips (fatigue) throughout the day.

3. Fats—The Good, the Bad, and the Ugly: It seems like everyone dreads fats, and we go to great lengths to avoid them. While it's true that we should watch our fat intake, avoiding fats completely is actually bad for our health.

Fats are an essential part of our diet. We need certain types of fats to aid in nerve development and brain function, and to make hormones. It's no wonder that people on low-fat diets can be so cranky! We should be getting approximately 25 percent of our daily calories from fats.

The Good: Essential Fatty Acids

Omega-3 and omega-6 fats are called essential fatty acids (EFAs) for two major reasons: they cannot be produced naturally by the body, so they must be ingested by way of food or supplements, and they are important for our immune system and brain function. Besides their health benefits, EFAs naturally make your hair more shiny. Great sources of EFAs include many of the foods that people avoid because "they're too high in fat," such as nuts, cold-water fish (salmon, sardines), soybeans, hemp oil, and seeds, including flax and chia.

Monounsaturated Fats

These help lower low-density lipoprotein (LDL) cholesterol (the bad one) while boosting high-density lipoprotein (HDL) cholesterol (the good one). They are safe for cooking at low temperatures, and food sources include olive oil, peanut oil, and canola oil.

Polyunsaturated Fats

Many health experts feel that polyunsaturated fats from whole food sources, which include nuts, seeds, vegetables, and whole grains, are better than saturated fats because they are cholesterol-free and come from plant foods. These fats are unstable and easily damaged by heat and processing, so they offer the best nutritional value when eaten raw; for instance, eat walnuts rather than use walnut oil.

The Bad (Maybe): Saturated Fats

What's all the fuss about saturated fats, the fats found mainly in animal foods, especially red meat, egg yolks, and butter, and also palm oil and coconut oil? They've been picked on for years as a major factor in the development of heart disease. However, natural health experts and forward thinkers have long suspected that saturated fats aren't as bad as we think they are; after all, before the oil refining process, most of our fats came from animal fats. Researchers too are now starting to change their tune about saturated fats. In 2010, the *American Journal of Clinical Nutrition* published two studies showing no significant evidence that dietary saturated fat is associated with an increased risk of heart disease. Dig deeper, and you'll find that it is unhealthy carbs that lead to heart disease, not saturated fat. Nonetheless, before you heat up the grill to make yourself a big, juicy steak, remember that *moderation is key*. In excess, saturated fats are not good for you.

The Ugly: Trans Fat

Foods containing trans fat, one of the most dangerous ingredients in our food supply, are a dime a dozen: margarine, cereals, granola bars, frozen pizza, fish sticks, puddings, peanut butter, chocolate bars, instant soup mixes, microwave popcorn, corn chips, pancake mixes, breaded foods, and

Sources of Fiber

- Lentils (½ cup, cooked), 8 g
- Frozen spinach (1 cup, cooked), 7 g
- Raspberries (½ cup, raw), 4 g
- Whole wheat bread (2 slices), 4 g
- Brown rice (1 cup, cooked), 3.5 g
- Almonds, dried (23 nuts, or 1 oz), 3.5 g
- Apple (medium with skin), 3.3 g
- Broccoli (½ cup, cooked), 2.5 g
- Carrots, raw (1 large), 2 g

more. They are hidden everywhere in processed foods, so *read labels carefully*! Keep an eye out for partially hydrogenated vegetable oil, margarine, and vegetable shortening.

4. Fiber—The Neglected Facilitator: There are two forms of fiber: soluble and insoluble. Soluble fiber is a soft fiber that helps control blood sugar and lower cholesterol. Oat bran, fruit, ground flax seeds, oatmeal, beans, lentils, and psyllium are excellent sources. Insoluble fiber (roughage) provides bulk to create larger, softer stools. Wheat bran, cereals, and skins of fruits and vegetables provide mainly insoluble fibers. It's important to include both in your diet daily.

Plant foods in their natural form—for example, a whole apple—provide fiber, whereas there is little or no fiber in animal products such as meat, poultry, fish, eggs, and dairy, or in refined grains such as white bread, white rice, and white pasta.

Ever wonder why fiber is so important?

- It creates volume in the stomach, causing you to feel full faster, and it cuts your appetite, preventing overeating.
- It helps prevent constipation and type 2 diabetes.
- It helps to reduce the risk of breast cancer, heart disease, and bowel disease, including irritable bowel syndrome (IBS), diverticulosis, diverticulitis, hemorrhoids, polyps, and colon cancer.
- It gently cleanses the colon and provides bulk for stools.
- Soluble fiber binds to cholesterol, fat, and toxins in your digestive system and removes them as part of your stool.

If your body functions best on a low-carb menu, supplemental fiber is available in many forms. Great options for fiber intake with foods are ground flax seed (or flax meal) and chia seeds, which can be sprinkled on yogurt and hot or cold cereal, added to a smoothie, or simply mixed with water.

5. Vitamins and Minerals—The Essential Elements: Many vitamins and minerals found in foods are lost when they are processed as packaged foods. Often a product will be advertised as vitamin or mineral enriched, but added nutrients are not always absorbed by the body as readily as nutrients from whole, natural foods.

Vitamins and Minerals with Funky Names

Ingredients such as pyridoxine hydrochloride, cyanocobalamin, and thiamine mononitrate sound like chemical additives, but they're not. These ingredients are actually nutrients that have been added to boost the nutritional content of a product. Here's a list of common nutrients with funky names that might be mistaken for additives.

Alpha-tocopherol: This may sound a little like a college fraternity, but it's a type of vitamin E. An antioxidant, vitamin E protects cell membranes and prolongs the life of red blood cells, the cells that deliver oxygen and nutrients to all the body's tissues. It's found naturally in seeds, oils, and some vegetables. The version d-alpha-tocopherol (you might see it listed as d-alpha-tocopherol acetate) is the natural and most biologically active form of vitamin E. The synthetic version, dl-alpha-tocopherol, is only half as effective as the natural form.

Ascorbic acid: This is simply good ol' vitamin C. A powerful antioxidant, ascorbic acid protects foods from oxidation. In the human body, vitamin C helps with iron absorption as well as collagen production to keep skin young and elastic. Natural sources include citrus, raw broccoli, red peppers, strawberries, and tomatoes.

Biotin: This member of the B family of vitamins assists the body in breaking down protein and carbohydrate molecules. Natural sources include yeast, liver, kidney, and eggs.

Calcium lactate: Calcium lactate is produced when lactic acid, an acid that exists in certain milk products, including yogurt, reacts with calcium carbonate. The result is white crystals that you find in milk and other dairy products. This is a highly absorbable form of calcium.

Copper gluconate: This absorbable form of copper can be used for a variety of ailments, including acne, the common cold, and high blood pressure. It is used in many nutritional supplements.

Choose Whole Grains

The terms *whole grain* and *multigrain* are not necessarily the same thing. *Whole grain* denotes that all three parts of the grain (the bran, the germ, and the endosperm) are present. While *multigrain* should mean that multiple whole grains are included, it can sometimes mean that more than one refined grain product is used. Since refined grains are no better than white bread, *choose a whole grain product* instead.

Savvy Tip: FIBER

When you're introducing a fiber supplement into your diet, begin with just ⅛ or ¼ teaspoon and increase gradually to the amount listed on the package. You may experience more gas and bloating at first, but once these symptoms go away and you are having more frequent bowel movements (an important key to good health), keep increasing your dosage slowly by ¼ or ½ teaspoon until you are going to the bathroom at least once or twice a day.

Cyanocobalamin: This is the technical term for vitamin B_{12}, which is essential for healthy red blood cells and helps maintain a healthy nervous system. It is found naturally in all animal foods and animal by-products such as milk, eggs, and yogurt.

d-Calcium pantothenate: Synthetically prepared from pantothenic acid and sold as a vitamin B_5 supplement. It's commonly added to foods and supplements, and is used to treat stress, morning stiffness and pain, as well as acne.

Ferrous fumarate: Also known as iron (II) fumarate, this form of iron helps to make hemoglobin, a protein in red blood cells that transports oxygen to all cells, and it also helps cells obtain energy.

Ferric orthophosphate: Another form of iron generally used to enrich bread, pasta, cereal, rice, syrup, animal feed, and other food products. It is added to foods because it is odorless and tasteless.

Magnesium oxide: This source of the mineral magnesium is used for indigestion, as an antacid, and as a short-term laxative.

Mixed tocopherols: See *alpha-tocopherol*.

Niacinamide: Also known as vitamin B_3, this form of niacin helps convert food to energy, supports the nervous system, and is needed for fat and protein metabolism. It is found naturally in whole grains, brewer's yeast, milk, meat, fish, eggs, and green vegetables.

Pantothenic acid: Vitamin B_5, pantothenic acid, is necessary for the formation of certain nerve-regulating substances. Natural sources include whole grains, eggs, kidney, peanuts, rice, and wheat bran.

Potassium iodide: This compound is formed by the combination of potassium and iodine and is represented by KI. Potassium is essential for the body's cells to function correctly. Iodine is a component of thyroid hormone, which is important for growth, development, and the regulation of the metabolic rate.

Pyridoxine hydrochloride: Vitamin B_6 promotes red blood cell production, is an essential part of amino acid production and breakdown, helps regulate hormones, assists the immune system, and has a variety of other functions in the body. It is found naturally in bread, meat, fish, eggs, beans, bananas, nuts, and seeds.

Riboflavin: Vitamin B_2, riboflavin, is needed for energy metabolism and for building and maintaining body tissues. It is found naturally in green vegetables, dairy, meat, fish, whole grains, and eggs.

Silicon dioxide: Also known as silica, this mineral is used as an anticaking agent in dairy products and products that contain whey, and in a wide range of products including some vegetables, pasta, and breakfast cereals. In the body, silica promotes the formation of connective tissue, so it's beneficial for healthy bones, skin, and hair.

Sodium selenite: This essential mineral is a salt and a source of the trace mineral selenium.

Thiamine hydrochloride: This synthetic form of vitamin B_1 is a crystalline substance used as a dietary supplement in foods, including enriched flour products, breakfast cereals, peanut butter, and skimmed milk.

Thiamine mononitrate: A form of vitamin B_1, this vitamin is needed for the production of adenosine triphosphate (ATP), a major energy source for the body. It is found naturally in whole grain breads and cereals.

Tocopherols: See *alpha-tocopherol.*

Tricalcium phosphate: This form of calcium is used in food and powdered spices as an anticaking agent. It is also used as a nutritional supplement. It occurs naturally in cow's milk.

Vitamin A palmitate: This is a synthetic form of vitamin A made with a combination of retinol (pure vitamin A) and palmitic acid (the acid found in palm oil). Natural sources of vitamin A include liver, eggs, butter, and fish.

Types of vitamins and minerals

Zinc oxide: This form of zinc is added to foods to enhance nutritional value. Zinc is needed for hundreds of functions, including carbohydrate digestion, prostate function, stomach acid production, and protein metabolism. Natural sources include meat, seafood, soybeans, spinach, egg yolk, and mushrooms.

Natural versus Organic

We are often asked what the difference is between *organic* and *natural*, and whether the terms are interchangeable. The short answer is they have very different meanings.

In reality, *natural* means very little. Food companies use it in a variety of ways, such as "made with natural ingredients," which could mean that just two of twenty ingredients are natural. The word *natural* in a product name or on the front of a package does not mean that it is 100 percent natural. Always read the ingredients; you'd be surprised how tricky some manufacturers can be. If you can understand all the ingredients listed, that is a good indication of how natural the product really is.

Organic products differ from natural in that *organic* refers to farming methods used to grow and process our food and fiber supply without the use of pesticides, herbicides, antibiotics, additives, growth hormones, or irradiation. Organic food is minimally processed, so fewer nutrients are lost; thus it maintains its wholesome value. In addition, organic food is not altered genetically—a process commonly referred to as genetic engineering or genetically modified organisms (GMOs).

GMOs: Unknown Risks

Genetically modified foods are everywhere, and you probably don't even know you're eating them. Proponents of genetically modified foods point to their many benefits: boosting agricultural production and potentially bringing an end to world hunger; decreased use of pesticides by creating

The Cost of Healthy Living

We know what you're thinking: healthy eating costs more. It's true, and no one is denying it. But when it comes right down to it, we're talking about your health and your children's health. Get this: 95 percent of money spent on health care in the United States goes toward treating illness, and only 5 percent is spent on prevention. Now, that's something to think about, isn't it?

Natural:
Presently, some consumers are pushing for stricter use of this term.

pest-resistant crops; and enhanced nutritional value by fortifying plants with additional nutrients. But critics warn of unknown and unpredictable health and environmental risks of new organisms that would never occur in nature.

Genetically modified foods are created by adding genes from bacteria, viruses, or animals to a plant's gene sequence to give it a desired trait, such as resistance to pests or to increase crop yield. These genetically modified seeds (and any other genetically modified life form) are called genetically modified organisms (GMOs). Genetically engineered (GE) food refers to any product containing or derived from GMOs.

The "big four" GMO ingredients are soybeans, corn, canola, and cotton. You may not think you eat a lot of soy or corn, but plenty of products are made from them, including corn syrup and soy lecithin. The fact is that soy, corn, and cotton are in everything from your cereal to your shampoo to the clothes that you wear. Because of the prevalence of these ingredients in everyday foods, experts estimate that 70 percent or more of processed or packaged foods contain GMOs.

The USDA does not currently require manufacturers to label GMO foods, so you wouldn't know the difference between a product made from a GMO and one made from an heirloom, or original variety, of corn or soy. If a food isn't labeled organic or non-GMO, look at the list of ingredients to identify any that are likely genetically modified. A few that you'll frequently find in many packaged foods are:

+ Canola oil
+ Corn oil
+ Cottonseed oil
+ High-fructose corn syrup
+ Soybean oil
+ Soy lecithin

For more information, visit www.naturallysavvy.com.

Fair Trade and Sustainability

Fair-trade products are grown with the planet and people in mind. Certifiers guarantee that fair-trade products such as cocoa, coffee, tea, rice, and sugar are grown in a sustainable manner; they also ensure that farmers are paid a fair price for their product and workers are treated fairly and earn a decent wage. Look for fair-trade logos on packages.

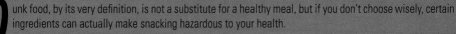

*J*unk food, by its very definition, is not a substitute for a healthy meal, but if you don't choose wisely, certain ingredients can actually make snacking hazardous to your health.

We've come up with our list of the "Worst Offenders," and we tell you why.

Trans Fat

Trans fat begins with partially hydrogenated oil. Hydrogenation is the chemical process that turns a liquid vegetable oil into solid fat. Trans fat is produced when oil is converted from liquid to solid form to produce a certain consistency and extend the shelf life of food.

These deadly fats are estimated to cause at least thirty thousand deaths each year. Trans fat not only increases the risk of heart attack by raising LDL and triglyceride (a type of fat in the bloodstream and fat tissue) levels but also has been linked to prostate cancer, breast cancer, Alzheimer's disease, diabetes, and obesity.

Zero Tolerance for Trans Fat

According to the FDA, Americans ingest an average of 5.8 grams of trans fat daily. This translates into 2,117 grams (almost 5 pounds) of trans fat per year.

How is it we are still eating that much trans fat if we are avoiding products that contain it? That's because foods that include less than 0.5 grams of trans fat per serving are allowed to state "0" trans fat on the Nutrition Facts panel. It doesn't mean the product does not contain any trans fat—it's a label loophole. If you see an ingredient listed as "partially hydrogenated" on a food label, avoid it because that means the product *does* contain trans fat. Bottom line: avoid it at all costs.

Sugar: Its Own Food Group?

Sugar has many forms: high-fructose corn syrup, fruit juice concentrate, evaporated cane juice, brown rice syrup, and words ending in -*ose* (glucose, dextrose, fructose, maltose, sucrose). It is important to read food labels carefully to clarify whether a product has hidden sources of sugar.

Warnings about sugar used to focus mainly on its causing dental cavities. People grew up thinking fat made people fat and sugar was relatively harmless. Back then, most meals were homemade and prepared from whole, natural ingredients. The story is very different now.

Sugar used to be called "white gold." Today it's considered "white poison." It creates imbalances in the human body, contributing to fatigue, blood sugar problems, intestinal problems (such as gas and encouraging the spread of unhealthy intestinal bacteria and fungi), and premenstrual syndrome (PMS).

According to the USDA, teenagers aged twelve to nineteen have the highest sweetener intake of any age group, at 137.4 pounds a year per person. This number includes sugar, corn syrup, and other sweeteners. That translates to 312 cups of sugar per year, or ¾ cup of sugar *per day*!

Teenage boys consume more sugar than girls and, surprisingly, adult males consume 25 percent more sugar than adult females. The problem isn't just the bevy of treats and soft drinks we consume (one can of soda alone has about 8 teaspoons of sugar) but also the concealed sources of sugar in processed foods. If you read labels carefully, you'll find sugar in ready-to-eat cereals, ketchup, milk products, canned foods, fruit-bottomed yogurt, salad dressings, crackers, breads, and even toothpaste.

Where Does Sugar Come From?

Most of the added sugar in our foods comes from sugarcane (80 percent) or sugar beet, a root vegetable (20 percent).

Sugarcane has been used to sweeten life for some three thousand years, but it's only recently that we've used technology to make refined sugar products. Long before white sugar, people would simply chew on sugarcane for a sweet treat, and in many Asian countries, you can still find fresh cut sugarcane in the market to satisfy your sweet tooth.

Sugar, by Many Other Names . . .

Until recently, all sugars were thought to be created equal. However, research is beginning to show that certain types of refined sugar, such as high-fructose corn syrup (mentioned throughout this book), may affect us more than other types.

High-fructose corn syrup (HFCS): This inexpensive substitute for real sugar is used primarily to sweeten beverages, including soft drinks. The American Heart Association identifies sugar-sweetened beverages as the main source of added sugars in the American diet, suggesting that liquid calories are more likely to lead to weight gain than calories obtained from solid foods. HFCS, made from yellow dent corn, is being shown to promote increased belly fat and insulin resistance—not to mention the long list of chronic diseases that result indirectly. The fructose in high-fructose corn syrup goes directly to your liver, where it converts to fat. The fat then gets sent to the bloodstream, resulting in elevated triglyceride levels, a risk factor for heart disease.

New research shows that fructose (like the fructose in HFCS) causes cancer cells to metastasize in a way that other sugars don't, proving that there is a difference between fructose and other sugars. All sugars can lead to health problems, but high-fructose corn syrup is worse in terms of cancer risk.

Less Processed Sugar

These forms of sugar are less processed than refined sugars and may be less likely to cause health problems:

- Agave (we recommend the brand Xagave [www.xagave.com], which contains only 49 percent fructose)
- Barley malt
- Brown rice syrup
- Date sugar
- Evaporated cane juice
- Honey
- Maple syrup
- Molasses
- Sucanat
- Turbinado

Not-So-Sweet Artificial Sweeteners

The FDA approves these artificial sweeteners for use in food:

- **Acesulfame potassium, or ace K (brand names, Sunett, Sweet One):** This calorie-free sweetener is two hundred times sweeter than sugar. Even though ace K has been approved by the FDA for consumption since 1988, to date the FDA has not required further testing, though early studies indicated that the additive may cause cancer in animals.

- **Aspartame (Equal, NutraSweet):** Aspartame has been implicated in producing a wide variety of symptoms related mostly to the nervous system, such as headaches, dizziness, mood changes, convulsions, and memory loss. Before your body can eliminate aspartame, it converts to formaldehyde (which is a carcinogen and used for embalming dead bodies). Found in more than five thousand products, this artificial ingredient has been the source of more complaints to the FDA than any other food additive.

- **Neotame:** Up to thirteen thousand times sweeter than sucrose (white sugar), it is similar to aspartame in composition but without an amino acid called phenylalanine; nonetheless, long-term health studies have not been conducted to ensure its safety.

- **Saccharin (Sweet'N Low):** The first commercial artificial sweetener, saccharin has been proven to cause cancer in animals and is a suspected human carcinogen. While saccharin hasn't been shown to cause cancer in humans, why would you want to ingest a substance that is an animal carcinogen?

- **Sucralose (Splenda):** Sucralose is six hundred times sweeter than sugar and has been tied to numerous adverse effects. In a Duke University study, male rats were fed a daily dose of Splenda over a period of twelve weeks. Splenda reduced the amount of healthy bacteria (including *Bifidobacteria bifidum* and lactobacilli) in the intestines by 50 percent and contributed to increased body weight. While this study was conducted on animals, sucralose may cause similar effects in humans.

Although they are FDA approved, these sweeteners are not without safety risks and are best avoided.

📖 *See the glossary for more information on sugar.*

Sodium

According to the American Heart Association, we consume an average of 3,435 milligrams of sodium a day. To keep your blood pressure in check, limit your daily sodium intake to 1,500 milligrams or less.

Your home cooking represents only 10 percent to 20 percent of your daily sodium intake. Adding table salt to your cooking or meals adds 5 percent to 10 percent, and 10 percent is found in plant and animal foods. Most (75 percent) of the sodium we consume comes from convenience foods, such as canned and processed foods, restaurant food, and fast food.

It may be difficult to control all the sodium in your diet—especially if you dine out or eat takeout regularly—but for what you can control, be sure to read labels. You can tell how much sodium a packaged food item contains by looking at its Nutrition Facts panel. The amount of sodium is listed clearly in milligrams, and the % Daily Value indicates the percentage of your maximum recommended daily intake. Read the ingredients list carefully and look for words such as: Sodium (or disodium) *anything,* including sodium benzoate, disodium inosinate, disodium guanylate, sodium caseinate, monosodium glutamate, sodium citrate, sodium phosphate, disodium phosphate, trisodium phosphate.

Food Additives

The Rainbow Connection: Artificial Colors

They're in our cereals, cosmetics, even in pharmaceutical drugs, and especially in candy. Almost all the popular brands of candy we reviewed were laced with artificial colors. Kids love those bright red, pink, yellow, orange,

Brown Sugar versus White Sugar

It's a common misconception that brown sugar is "healthier" or "more natural" than white table sugar. In reality, brown sugar is just white sugar with a bit of molasses added.

Artificial Color: Dye versus Lake

The FDA categorizes artificial color additives as either dyes or lakes.

- **Dyes** dissolve in water and can be used in beverages, dry mixes, baked goods, confections, dairy products, pet foods, and a variety of other products.

- **Lakes** are the insoluble form of the dye. More stable than dyes, lakes are ideal for coloring products containing fats and oils, such as hard candies, chewing gums, cakes, and mixes.

Dye or lake, we suggest you avoid all artificial colors.

Read more about artificial colors in the glossary.

green, and blue hues, but their little bodies don't. Most artificial dyes have been linked to hyperactivity, attention deficit disorder (ADD), and attention deficit/hyperactivity disorder (ADHD).

Parents and pediatricians have been complaining about artificial colors in food for more than forty years, and their concerns have been largely disregarded. Finally, in 2004, an analysis of fifteen studies found evidence that artificial colors worsen the behavior of children with ADHD. Two more studies then found that artificial dyes do, in fact, affect the behavior of children without behavioral disorders.

All food and drink labels must list the additives they contain, including artificial colors. The FDA, which assigns FD&C (Federal Food, Drug, and Cosmetic) numbers to artificial dyes, approves colors for use in food.

Natural Food Colorings

Use of natural food dyes is skyrocketing, in part due to consumer concern over the synthetic versions. Look for products that contain natural dyes, including:

- Beet juice
- Beta-carotene
- Grape skin extract
- Paprika oleoresin
- Fruit and vegetable juices
- Saffron

The food dyes listed below are derived from natural sources and thus are considered natural; however, they have been linked with allergic reactions and should be avoided by those who are sensitive:

- Annatto extract
- Caramel
- Cochineal extract or carmine

Artificial Flavors

When "artificial flavors" is listed on a label, it is a blanket term that could include one or hundreds of unnatural additives. For example, a typical artificial strawberry flavor contains forty-nine chemical ingredients!

Monosodium glutamate: This artificial flavor is found in thousands of different processed foods such as fast food, chips, flavored rice, and soup. Even though the FDA classifies the flavoring as "Generally Recognized as Safe," or GRAS, it has received many consumer complaints about adverse reactions to foods containing MSG. Some of these reactions include sweating, facial numbness, heart palpitations, nausea, and weakness.

Preservatives and Emulsifiers

Hundreds of preservatives and emulsifiers (used to bind ingredients together) are added to processed foods. Not all are dangerous, but do your best to avoid these.

BHA (butylated hydroxyanisole) and BHT (butylated hydroxytoluene): These two closely related preservatives are added to foods containing fats and oils to prevent oxidation, slow rancidity, and prolong shelf life. They have been known to impair kidney and liver function, and the US Department of Health and Human Services National Toxicology Program lists BHA as a possible carcinogen.

For more information on additives, visit www.naturallysavvy.com.

Polysorbate 80: This additive is commonly used as an emulsifier in foods such as ice cream. It's been shown to affect the immune system and has caused severe anaphylactic shock, a potentially fatal allergic reaction. Numerous animal studies have also linked polysorbate 80 to infertility.

Potassium sorbate: This preservative is used to extend the shelf life of a product by inhibiting the growth of yeasts and molds. This way, a convenience store can stock a food for years without worrying about it going bad. Although potassium sorbate is considered to be safe, sorbates have been linked to asthma, skin rashes, diarrhea, and hyperactivity in some sensitive people.

Propionates: These preservatives, including sodium propionate, are added to food and baked goods to inhibit the growth of microbes, such as bacteria and protozoa. Some people report having experienced migraines, headaches, and gastrointestinal complaints after ingesting them.

Sodium benzoate: This preservative is often added to acidic foods and drinks. It is linked to allergic reactions and is a carcinogen.

Sulfur dioxide: This falls under the category of sulfites, a group of preservatives commonly used for dried fruit, wine, flavored vinegars (balsamic), salad dressings, sausages, and some potato products. Sulfites are a common allergen and can cause headaches, bowel irritability, behavioral problems, skin rashes, and other symptoms. They are particularly dangerous for asthmatic individuals, who can develop bronchospasm (a sudden constriction of the airways) after eating foods or drinking wine preserved with sulfur dioxide or other sulfur preservatives.

TBHQ (tertiary butylhydroquinone): TBHQ is a petroleum-based food additive used to increase the shelf life of products and prevent rancidity of fats. It has been associated with nausea, vomiting, and tinnitus, and prolonged exposure has been linked with cancer.

WORST INGREDIENTS CHART

For a printable version of this list, visit: www.naturallysavvy.com.

We came up with a list of the 'worst ingredients' commonly found in junk food. Keep a copy of this list handy to help you make more mindful choices whenever you are grocery shopping. The list is divided into two parts:

> **Red: Worst Ingredients** *(should be strictly avoided)*
> **Yellow: Also Beware of** *(should be used with caution)*

Below are the worst ingredients we found in the products included in this book.

Red: Worst Ingredients

- Acesulfame potassium, ace-K *(artificial sweetener)*
- Artificial butter flavor *(artificial flavor)*
- Artificial color
- Artificial flavor
- Artificial raspberry flavor *(artificial flavor)*
- Artificial strawberry flavor *(artificial flavor)*
- Aspartame *(artificial sweetener)*
- BHA *(preservative)*
- BHT *(preservative)*
- Blue 1 and blue 1 lake *(artificial colors)*
- Blue 2 and Blue 2 lake *(artificial colors)*
- Green color *(artificial color)*
- High-fructose corn syrup *(sweetener)*
- Monosodium glutamate (MSG) *(flavor enhancer)*
- Neotame *(artificial sweetener)*
- Olestra, Olean *(fat substitute)*

- Partially hydrogenated cottonseed, palm, palm kernel, soybean, and vegetable oil *(trans fats)*
- Partially hydrogenated lard *(trans fat)*
- Polysorbate 60 *(emulsifier)*
- Polysorbate 65 *(emulsifier)*
- Polysorbate 80 *(emulsifier)*
- Preservatives
- Red 3 *(artificial color)*
- Red 40 and Red 40 lake *(artificial colors)*
- Sodium benzoate *(preservative)*
- Sodium metabisulfite *(preservative, antioxidant)*
- Sodium nitrite *(preservative)*
- Sucralose *(artificial sweetener)*
- Sulfur dioxide *(preservative, antioxidant)*
- TBHQ *(preservative, antioxidant)*
- Yellow 5 and Yellow 5 lake *(artificial colors)*
- Yellow 6 and Yellow 6 lake *(artificial colors)*

Unjunk Your Junk Food

Yellow: Also Beware of

- Annatto, Annatto extract *(natural color)*
- Artificial vanilla flavor *(artificial flavor)*
- Autolyzed yeast *(flavor enhancer)*
- Autolyzed yeast extract *(flavor enhancer)*
- Benzoic acid *(preservative)*
- Caffeine
- Calcium disodium (EDTA) *(preservative, stabilizer)*
- Ethylenediaminetetraacetic acid (EDTA) *(preservative, stabilizer)*
- Caramel color *(natural color)*
- Carrageenan *(emulsifier)*
- Coffee
- Diacetyl tartaric acid ester of monoglyceride (DATEM) *(emulsifier)*
- Disodium guanylate *(flavor enhancer)*
- Disodium inosinate *(flavor enhancer)*
- Ester of rosin *(emulsifier)*
- Glucono delta-lactone *(stabilizer)*
- Glyceryl tripropionine *(emulsifier)*
- Hydrogenated canola, coconut, cottonseed, palm, palm kernel, rapeseed, and soybean oils *(potential trans fat sources)*
- Hydrolyzed milk protein, hydrolyzed protein *(flavor enhancer)*
- Margarine *(potential trans fat source)*
- Polyglycerol polyricinoleate (PGPR) *(emulsifier)*
- Potassium sorbate *(preservative)*
- Propylene glycol *(emulsifier)*
- Sodium carboxymethylcellulose *(thickener, stabilizer)*
- Sodium caseinate *(emulsifier, stabilizer)*
- Sodium hexametaphosphate *(stabilizer)*
- Sodium propionate *(antimicrobial agent, preservative)*
- Sodium stearoyl lactylate *(emulsifier, dough conditioner)*
- Sorbitan monostearate *(emulsifier, stabilizer)*
- Titanium dioxide *(artificial color)*
- Vanillin *(flavoring agent)*
- Vegetable oil shortening *(potential trans fat source)*
- Vegetable shortening *(potential trans fat source)*
- Yeast extract *(flavor enhancer)*

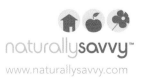

naturallysavvy™

chips, dips & party foods

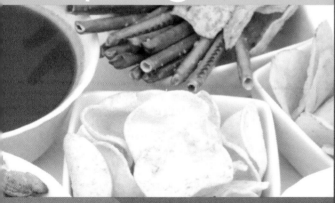

We Just Can't Get Enough of Our Salt

Chips, nachos, and popcorn make the ideal party foods; they're easy to share, great for casual snacking, and the perfect finger foods. It's no wonder more than 99 percent of American homes purchase salty snacks, and potato chip sales exceed 2.8 billion annually!

savvy tip

Potato chip ingredients should be simple: POTATOES + OIL + SALT. But some seasoned varieties may contain flavor enhancers—some natural, some not. Many companies, including Frito-Lay, have committed to removing unhealthy additives such as MSG, artificial colors and flavors from their products. This is in response to consumers' appeals for "cleaner labels." That's a change we like.

WORST INGREDIENTS

we found in salty snacks

- Artificial colors
- Artificial flavors
- Monosodium glutamate (MSG)
- Olestra
- Partially hydrogenated oils (trans fats)
- TBHQ

also beware of

- Annatto color
- Autolyzed yeast extract
- Disodium guanylate
- Disodium inosinate
- Glyceryl tripropionine
- Sodium caseinate
- Potassium sorbate
- Yeast extract

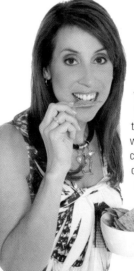

MISLEADING MARKETING

You'll often see bags of chips marked "cholesterol free," but it's not like the manufacturer did anything to remove cholesterol—it was never there to begin with. Most potato chips don't have cholesterol because they're cooked in unsaturated vegetable oils, which are naturally cholesterol free. The only potato chips with cholesterol are flavored and contain dairy, such as chips with cheddar cheese or sour cream.

Reasons You Might Be Craving
. . . Salty Snacks

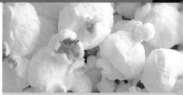

LOW THYROID FUNCTION
People with low thyroid function might yearn for salty foods, but their bodies are, in fact, in need of iodine, a mineral in salt. Other symptoms might include cold hands, feeling tired, and difficulty losing weight. Consult your doctor if you are experiencing these symptoms.

ADRENAL FATIGUE
Low adrenal function can cause salt cravings. If you lie wide-awake at three o'clock in the morning and have symptoms of depression, speak to your doctor about testing your adrenal hormone levels—produced by the glands located above each kidney—via a simple blood or saliva test.

LOW IRON
Craving salty foods may also be a symptom of iron deficiency. A simple blood test can identify if iron-deficiency anemia (a shortage of red blood cells in the circulation) is the cause or a factor in your fatigue.

Olestra Is **Bad** News

Some brands of fat-free snacks contain olestra (Olean), a fat substitute that prevents fats—and, unfortunately, important fat-soluble nutrients—from being absorbed. The FDA approved olestra in 1996 but required food labels to state: "This product contains olestra. Olestra may cause abdominal cramping and loose stools. Olestra inhibits the absorption of some vitamins and other nutrients. Vitamins A, D, E, and K have been added." They lifted the label warning requirement in 2003 based on research from Procter & Gamble, makers of olestra. Talk about letting the fox guard the henhouse.

fact

A potato naturally has thirty to fifty times more potassium than sodium, approximately 125 calories, and very little fat.

healthy tip

If you have chronically high blood pressure, or hypertension, make sure your diet includes more potassium than sodium. A 2009 study showed that people with a low-sodium, high-potassium diet are less likely to experience heart disease and stroke. Fruits and vegetables are naturally high in potassium and low in sodium, important for maintaining normal blood pressure, and can be helpful for lowering elevated blood pressure. Potassium is found in most raw fruits and vegetables, including bananas and potatoes, as well as in yogurt.

fried potato chips

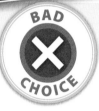

Great Value Potato Chips
Sour Cream & Onion (Walmart Brand)

Monosodium glutamate (MSG)

Many people associate MSG with Chinese food, but MSG is found in thousands of different processed foods that we eat on a regular basis such as fast food, chips, flavored rice, and soup.

Artificial flavors

Food processing techniques cause foods and natural ingredients to lose much of their flavor, creating a dependence on artificial flavors. The American flavor industry now has annual revenues of $1.4 billion! This product states "Artificially Flavored" right on the front of the package.

Glyceryl tripropionine

A plasticizer, or additive that increases the pliability of the substance to which it's added.

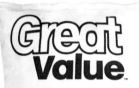

Nutrition Facts
Serving size About 12 chips (1 oz/28 g)

Calories 150	Calories from fat 90
Total fat 9 g	
Saturated fat 1 g	
Trans fat 0 g	
Cholesterol 0 mg	
Sodium 210 mg	
Total carbohydrates 16 g	
Dietary fiber 1 g	
Sugars 1 g	
Protein 2 g	

INGREDIENTS: potatoes, sunflower oil and/or corn oil, sour cream and onion seasoning (nonfat dry milk, maltodextrin, whey powder, onion powder, salt, sour cream powder [sour cream {milk ingredients, bacterial culture}, citric acid], dextrose, monosodium glutamate, dehydrated parsley, lactose, natural and artificial flavors [maltodextrin, milk, starter distillate, natural flavor, glyceryl tripropionine, modified cornstarch, citric acid, artificial flavor, modified cellulose], sunflower oil, silicon dioxide, whey protein concentrate, buttermilk powder, citric acid, sodium caseinate), salt.

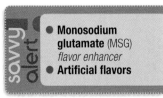

savvy alert
- **Monosodium glutamate** (MSG) *flavor enhancer*
- **Artificial flavors**

savvy serving

Mindlessly knocking back a whole bag of potato chips is equivalent to eating *five* servings. That's 750 calories and 40 grams of fat! Measure your portion size according to the package before you snack.

Kettle Brand Potato Chips
Sour Cream and Onion

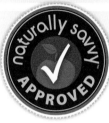

Nutrition Facts
Serving size 13 chips (1 oz/28 g)

Calories 150	Calories from fat 80

Total fat 9 g
Saturated fat 1 g
Trans fat 0 g
Cholesterol 0 mg
Sodium 140 mg
Total carbohydrates 16 g
Dietary fiber Less than 1 g
Sugars 1 g
Protein 2 g

INGREDIENTS: potatoes, vegetable oil (safflower and/or sunflower oil), yogurt powder (whey, nonfat milk), nonfat dry milk, salt, dried onion, dried cane syrup, dried sour cream (cultured cream, nonfat milk), dried parsley, dried garlic, turmeric, lactic acid, citric acid.

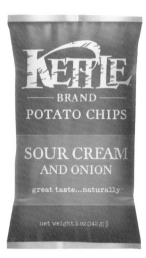

Savvy Pick
Both brands have the same calories and fat, but Kettle has less sodium than Walmart's Great Value brand and no MSG. For that reason, Kettle gets our Naturally Savvy Seal of Approval™.

Honorable Mention
✦ Route 11 Potato Chips
Sour Cream & Chive

What is ...?

Glutamate

Glutamate, an amino acid, occurs naturally in many foods, but it's also a component of MSG. The problem arises when flavor-enhancing compounds called free glutamates are added to foods. They act as excitatory neurotransmitters, causing the nerves in your brain to fire rapidly and repeatedly. While this stimulation heightens our sense of taste, it also can cause a variety of symptoms, including impaired memory, perception, cognition, and motor skills.

baked potato crisps

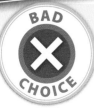

Herr's
Baked Potato Crisps — Cheddar & Sour Cream

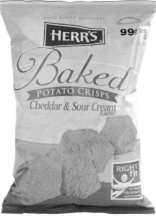

Monosodium glutamate (MSG)

When researchers fed MSG to animals in a laboratory study, the animals ate twice as much. The researchers concluded that MSG consumption was very likely to damage the brain's ability to regulate appetite.

Feingold Program on Additives

The late San Francisco pediatrician and allergist, Dr. Ben Feingold, developed the Feingold diet after he noticed that his patients reacted negatively—both physically and behaviorally—to some foods and food additives. To identify whether or not certain additives contribute to behavioral problems, the Feingold program eliminates:

✤ Artificial colors
✤ Artificial flavors
✤ Most artificial sweeteners
✤ The artificial preservatives BHA, BHT, and TBHQ

Nutrition Facts

Serving size About 13 crisps (1 bag/28.4 g)

Calories 120	Calories from fat 30
Total fat 3 g	
Saturated fat 0.5 g	
Trans fat 0 g	
Cholesterol 0 mg	
Sodium 330 mg	
Total carbohydrates 22 g	
Dietary fiber 2 g	
Sugars 2 g	
Protein 2 g	

INGREDIENTS: dehydrated potato flakes, modified corn starch, high-oleic sunflower and/or corn oil, sugar, salt, whey, maltodextrin, leavening (baking powder, monocalcium phosphate), canola oil, lecithin, dextrose, monosodium glutamate, cheddar cheese (cultured milk, salt enzymes), onion powder, sour cream (cultured cream, nonfat dry milk), whey protein concentrate, nonfat dry milk, natural and artificial flavors, disodium phosphate, citric acid, garlic powder, color (including Yellow 5, Yellow 6, and annatto), and lactic acid).

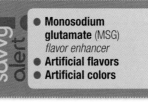

savvy alert

● **Monosodium glutamate** (MSG) *flavor enhancer*
● **Artificial flavors**
● **Artificial colors**

portion control

The problem with baked chips is that they give the illusion that since they are not fried, they are a healthy snack to be eaten with abandon. Remember, they are still a treat and contain quite a bit of sodium.

Michael Season's
Baked Potato Crisps—Cheddar & Sour Cream

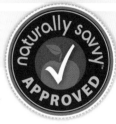

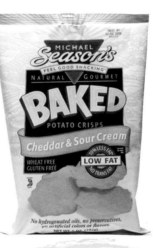

Nutrition Facts
Serving size 14 crisps (1 oz/28 g)

Calories 120	Calories from fat 25
Total fat 3 g	
Saturated fat 0.5 g	
Trans fat 0 g	
Cholesterol 0 mg	
Sodium 210 mg	
Total carbohydrates 21 g	
Dietary fiber 2 g	
Sugars 3 g	
Protein 2 g	

INGREDIENTS: dehydrated potatoes, modified food starch, sugar, sunflower oil, soy lecithin, leavening (monocalcium phosphate, sodium bicarbonate), and seasoning consisting of rice flour, salt, palm oil, dried sour cream (cultured cream, nonmilk), corn syrup solids, cheddar cheese (pasteurized milk, cheese cultures, salt, enzymes), natural flavors, maltodextrin, onion powder, whey, sodium caseinate, buttermilk, butter (cream, salt), garlic powder, lactic acid, citric acid, paprika extract (color), dipotassium phosphate, yeast extract, disodium phosphate, canola oil, natural smoke flavor.

Savvy Pick

With the same calories and fat as Herr's, but with 120 milligrams less sodium, no artificial colors, and no MSG (although it does contain yeast extract and sodium caseinate, both which can cause reactions similar to MSG in some people), Michael Season's is the better choice of the two brands.

Yeast Extract

This flavor-enhancing additive contains free glutamic acid, a component of MSG, but is less concentrated. Also, its extracting process is less harsh, in that it doesn't require the use of chemicals the way MSG does. In some cases, manufacturers add MSG to yeast extract; but even if they don't, you may still have a reaction to foods containing yeast extract, since it is a form of free glutamic acid.

low-fat/light potato chips

BAD ✗ **CHOICE**

Lay's
Light Original Potato Chips—Fat Free

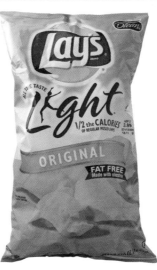

Did you know?
Products containing olestra are not actually fat free—rather, olestra is a synthetic ingredient that the body cannot absorb. Instead it is eliminated with your stool.

Fat-free flop
Olestra may inhibit the body's ability to absorb beneficial fat-soluble nutrients, including lycopene, lutein, and beta-carotene. In one study, only 8 grams of olestra per day (the amount you'd ingest from eating 16 potato chips containing olestra) for eight weeks caused a dramatic depletion of important carotenoids and fat-soluble vitamins.

Nutrition Facts
Serving size 1 oz/28 g

Calories 75	Calories from fat 0
Total fat 0 g	
Saturated fat 0 g	
Trans fat 0 g	
Cholesterol 0 mg	
Sodium 200 mg	
Total carbohydrates 17 g	
Dietary fiber 1 g	
Sugars 0 g	
Protein 2 g	

INGREDIENTS: potatoes, olestra, salt, alpha-tocopherol acetate (vitamin E), vitamin A palmitate, tocopherols (to protect flavor), vitamin K, vitamin D.

savvy alert
● **Olestra**

misleading marketing

The word *Lite* on a label implies the product is low in calories, but it may be referring instead to the color, flavor, or texture. Read the Nutrition Facts panel and the small print on the package carefully to determine what "lite" really means.

Brothers
All-Natural Potato Crisps—100% Fat Free

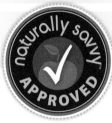

Nutrition Facts
Serving size 1 bag (0.85 oz/24 g)

Calories 35	Calories from fat 0

Total fat 0 g
   Saturated fat 0 g
   Trans fat 0 g
Cholesterol 0 mg
Sodium 260 mg
Total carbohydrates 8 g
   Dietary fiber 1 g
   Sugars 1 g
Protein 2 g

INGREDIENTS: fresh potatoes, sea salt.

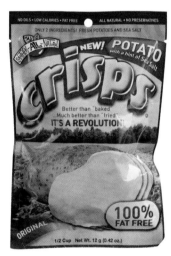

Savvy Pick
Talk about simplicity, Brothers All-Natural potato crisps' ingredients list can't be beat: just potatoes and sea salt. While Brothers does have more sodium than Lay's, it contains fewer calories and no olestra. These chips should receive many encores in your shopping cart.

Sea ⟶ VERSUS ⟵ Table
SALT

Table salt is composed of sodium chloride (the chemical name for table salt) and added iodine. Sea salt, on the other hand, is evaporated sea water and contains dozens of minerals from the ocean. White sea salt has been washed, so as a result some of the minerals have been washed away. **Best types:** gray, pink, or black sea salt. Himalayan salt is another good alternative, and all varieties are great for cooking. Try the brands Real Salt (Redmond Trading Co.) and Selina Naturally Celtic Sea Salt.

microwave popcorn—butter

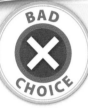

Orville Redenbacher's
Gourmet Popping Corn—Butter

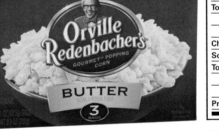

Diacetyl
Popcorn flavoring contains diacetyl, the chemical which gives popcorn its buttery flavor. Though it was approved by the FDA as a flavor ingredient, diacetyl may be hazardous when heated and inhaled over a long period of time. ConAgra, the nation's largest microwave popcorn maker and manufacturer (and makers of Act II and Orville Redenbacher brands) stopped using diacetyl in 2007.

GMO corn
A study found that genetically modified corn caused organ damage in rats, affecting kidney and liver function in particular. To avoid GMO corn, look for products that use organic corn or state "non-GMO corn" on the package.

Nutrition Facts
Serving size 1 cup, popped

Calories 30	Calories from fat 20
Total fat 2 g	
Saturated fat 1 g	
Trans fat 0 g	
Cholesterol 0 mg	
Sodium 40 mg	
Total carbohydrates 3 g	
Dietary fiber Less than 1 g	
Sugars Not available	
Protein 2 g	

INGREDIENTS: popping corn, palm oil, less than 2 percent of each of: salt, potassium chloride, butter, natural and artificial flavor, artificial color, TBHQ, and citric acid (for freshness).

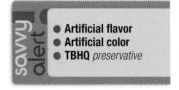

savvy alert
- Artificial flavor
- Artificial color
- TBHQ *preservative*

popcorn portion control Plain popcorn is naturally low in calories, but it's the toppings that tip the scale. One tablespoon of butter provides 100 calories and 11 grams of fat. A heart-healthy option is to drizzle extra-virgin olive oil or coconut oil over freshly popped corn and sprinkle some nutritional yeast flakes for a cheesy flavor and B vitamins.

Newman's Own Organics
Butter Flavored Pop's Corn

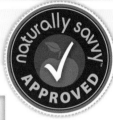

Nutrition Facts

Serving size 2.8 cups (28 g)

Calories 123	Calories from fat 42
	(44 calories for 1 cup)
Total fat 5 g	(1.8 grams for 1 cup)
Saturated fat 2 g	(0.7 grams for 1 cup)
Trans fat 0 g	
Cholesterol 0 mg	
Sodium 187 mg	(66 mg for 1 cup)
Total carbohydrates 17 g	(6 grams for 1 cup)
Dietary fiber 4 g	(1.4 grams for 1 cup)
Sugars 1 g	(0.36 grams for 1 cup)
Protein 3 g	(1 gram for 1 cup)

INGREDIENTS: organic popcorn, organic palm oil, natural buttter flavor (contains milk), salt, vitamin E (to preserve freshness).

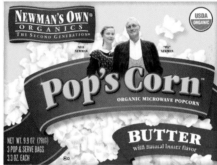

Savvy Pick
Newman's Own Organics Pop's Corn has more calories per one cup serving than Orville Redenbacher's plus more sodium, but we still prefer this brand since it is free of artificial ingredients such as artificial color.

Honorable Mention
❖ Orville Redenbacher's
Natural Line

What is ... PFOA

Perfluorooctanoic acid is a chemical used to coat the bags of microwavable popcorn and is used to make Teflon. It has been linked to ADHD in humans and cancer and infertility in animals. On average, Americans have 3 to 4 nanograms of PFOA per milliliter of blood.

DuPont, maker of Teflon, was fined for failing to report the health risks of PFOA, and the company has since vowed to eliminate the harmful chemical by 2015. Both Newman's Own Organics and Orville Redenbacher's say their bags are PFOA free.

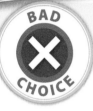

BAD X **CHOICE**

Doritos
Nacho Cheese

Sad truth

Sorry to disappoint you, Doritos lovers, but this product has such a long list of ingredients, many of which are red flags. The fact that it is still one of America's favorite snacks is just more evidence that either we aren't reading ingredient labels or we are choosing to ignore dangerous ingredients for the sake of taste.

Uber-long ingredients list

Dorito's ingredients list is so long, we had a hard time fitting it on one page so we had to shrink the font.

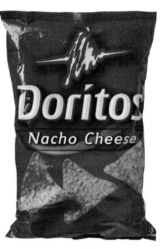

Nutrition Facts
Serving size About 11 chips (1 oz/28 g)

Calories 150	Calories from fat 70

Total fat 8 g

Saturated fat 1.5 g

Trans fat 0 g

Cholesterol 0 mg

Sodium 180 mg

Total carbohydrates 17 g

Dietary fiber 1 g

Sugars 1 g

Protein 2 g

INGREDIENTS: Whole corn, vegetable oil (contains one or more of the following: corn, soybean, and/or sunflower oil), salt, cheddar cheese (milk, cheese cultures, salt, enzymes), maltodextrin, wheat flour, whey, monosodium glutamate, buttermilk solids, Romano cheese from cow's milk (part-skim cow's milk, cheese cultures, salt, enzymes), whey protein concentrate, onion powder, partially hydrogenated soybean and cottonseed oil, corn flour, disodium phosphate, lactose, natural and artificial flavor, dextrose, tomato powder, spices, lactic acid, artificial color (including yellow 6, yellow 5, red 40), citric acid, sugar, garlic powder, red and green bell pepper powder, sodium caseinate, disodium inosinate, disodium guanylate, nonfat milk solids, whey protein isolate, and corn syrup solids.

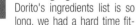

savvy alert

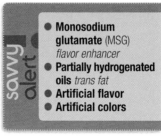

- **Monosodium glutamate** (MSG) *flavor enhancer*
- **Partially hydrogenated oils** *trans fat*
- **Artificial flavor**
- **Artificial colors**

calorie counting

One meal or snack will not cause you to gain weight. It takes 3,500 extra calories to "create" 1 pound of body fat. An extra cookie here, a few potato chips there . . . weight gain often occurs insidiously and over a period of time.

Garden of Eatin'
Organic Nacho Cheese

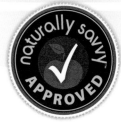

Nutrition Facts
Serving size 10 chips (1 oz)

Calories 140	Calories from fat 50
Total fat 6 g	
Saturated fat 0.5 g	
Trans fat 0 g	
Cholesterol 0 mg	
Sodium 140 mg	
Total carbohydrates 18 g	
Dietary fiber 2 g	
Sugars Less than 1 g	
Protein 2 g	

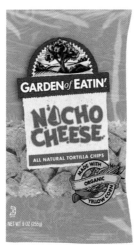

NET WT 9 OZ (255g)

INGREDIENTS: organic yellow corn, expeller-pressed safflower oil and/or canola oil and/or sunflower oil, organic cheddar cheese (milk) powder (organic cheddar cheese base [organic cheddar cheese, organic whey powder, lactic acid, disodium phosphate, annatto, natural flavor, enzymes], salt, organic whey, organic tomato powder, organic onion powder, organic autolyzed yeast extract, citric acid, organic mustard powder, organic garlic powder, organic cayenne pepper powder).

Savvy Pick
Doritos are a huge favorite, but trans fat, MSG, artificial colors, and artificial flavors all in one bag put Doritos among the worst offenders in this chapter! Garden of Eatin' Organic Nacho Cheese Tortilla Chips contain autolyzed yeast extract, which can cause reactions in some people (yes, even if it is organic), but let's face it: the ingredients list is a giant step up from Doritos. To add insult to injury, Doritos are higher in calories, fat, and sodium. Need we say more?

Honorable Mention
✦ Kettle Brand Tias!
   Nacho cheddar

savvy FACT
After evaluating the most popular brands of plain and multigrain tortilla chips, we found the ingredients to be relatively clean, with the major ingredients being corn, vegetable oil, and salt. The biggest difference is that the natural varieties use organic, non-GMO corn.

cheese puffs

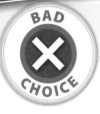

Cheetos
Cheese Puffs—Cheddar

Artificial color

If the food you are eating stains your fingers like Cheetos does it is a good indication that it may contain artificial colors.

Partially hydrogenated oils *trans fats*

A study on monkeys showed that diets containing trans fat are more likely to cause abdominal weight gain than diets containing the same amount of calories without the bad fats.

Monosodium glutamate (MSG)

The FDA has identified a condition dubbed MSG symptom complex, which can cause headaches, numbness, and weakness, and may temporarily exacerbate symptoms in those with severe asthma.

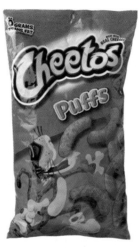

Nutrition Facts

Serving size About 13 chips (1 oz/28 g)

Calories 160	Calories from fat 90
Total fat 10 g	
Saturated fat 1.5 g	
Trans fat 0 g	
Cholesterol 0 g	
Sodium 370 mg	
Total carbohydrates 15 g	
Dietary fiber 0 g	
Sugars Less than 1 g	
Protein 2 g	

INGREDIENTS: enriched cornmeal (cornmeal, ferrous sulfate, niacin, thiamine mononitrate, riboflavin, and folic acid), vegetable oil (contains one of more of the following: corn, soybean, and/or sunflower oil, whey, salt, cheddar cheese [cultured milk, salt, enzymes], less than 2 percent each of partially hydrogenated soybean oil, maltodextrin, disodium phosphate, sour cream [cultured cream, nonfat milk], artificial flavor, monosodium glutamate, lactic acid, artificial color [including Yellow 6], citric acid).

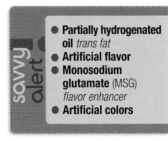

savvy alert
- **Partially hydrogenated oil** *trans fat*
- **Artificial flavor**
- **Monosodium glutamate** (MSG) *flavor enhancer*
- **Artificial colors**

Barbara's
Cheez Puff Bakes Original—Cheddar

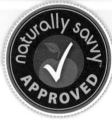

Nutrition Facts
Serving size About 1½ cups (1 oz/28 g)

Calories 150	Calories from fat 90
Total fat 10 g	
Saturated fat 2 g	
Trans fat 0 g	
Cholesterol 5 mg	
Sodium 200 mg	
Total carbohydrates 14 g	
Dietary fiber 1 g	
Sugars 1 g	
Protein 2 g	

INGREDIENTS: yellow cornmeal, expeller-pressed high-oleic (canola, sunflower, or safflower) oil, aged cheddar and blue cheese (pasteurized milk, salt, annatto extract, cheese cultures, natural enzymes), whey (milk), buttermilk solids, salt, lactic acid, paprika and turmeric extracts.

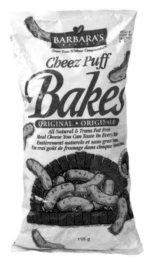

Savvy Pick
The fat and calories are similar in both products, but Cheetos has a lot more sodium, and has trans fat, MSG, and artificial colors—which give the cheese puffs their familiar orange color.

Honorable Mention
❖ Kudos to Cheetos for offering consumers a cleaner option with their *Natural White Cheddar Puffs*, made with organic cornmeal, real cheese, and no trans fat or MSG.

WEIGHTY MATTERS
WEIGHTY MATTERS

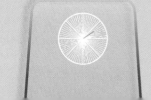

Serving sizes vary from product to product. If a product's label doesn't spell out the portion size for you—usually the number of chips per serving—then pull out your handy kitchen scale and weigh away.

dips—ranch dip

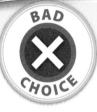

BAD CHOICE

Hidden Valley
Original Ranch Dip

Monosodium glutamate (MSG)

The Japanese company, Ajinomoto Co., Inc., the company that makes 33% of the world's MSG, is also the largest producer of aspartame.

A savvy tip about a double dip

If you ever wondered why double dipping is socially frowned upon, a microbiologist found that three to six double dips transfer about ten thousand bacteria from the eater's mouth to the communal bowl of dip. You had better think twice (but not dip twice) the next time you reach for a veggie to dip at a party.

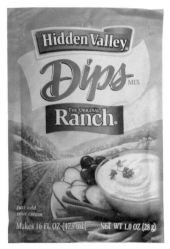

Nutrition Facts
Serving size 1.8 g

Calories 5	Calories from fat 0
Total fat 0 g	
Saturated fat 0 g	
Trans fat 0 g	
Cholesterol 0 mg	
Sodium 240 mg	
Total carbohydrates 1 g	
Dietary fiber 0 g	
Sugars 0 g	
Protein 0 g	

INGREDIENTS: maltodextrin, salt, monosodium glutamate, dried onion, dried garlic, spices, modified food starch, less than 2% of: buttermilk, calcium stearate, natural flavor (soy).

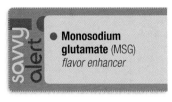

savvy alert

● **Monosodium glutamate** (MSG)
flavor enhancer

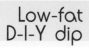

Low-fat D-I-Y dip

It's not hard to mimic the creamy texture of sour cream by substituting a low-fat, unflavored Greek yogurt. Two brands we really like are Oikos and Fage. Mix with caramelized onions and/or fresh herbs for a low-fat, great-tasting chip dip.

Simply Organic
Ranch Dip Mix

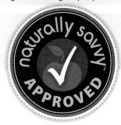

Nutrition Facts

Serving size 2 tsp (2.5 g)

Calories 10	Calories from fat 0
Total fat 0 g	
Saturated fat 0 g	
Trans fat 0 g	
Cholesterol 0 mg	
Sodium 150 mg	
Total carbohydrates 1 g	
Dietary fiber 0 g	
Sugars 1 g	
Protein 1 g	

INGREDIENTS: organic nonfat milk, sea salt, organic cane sugar, organic garlic, organic onion, organic carrot powder, organic celery seed, xanthan gum, organic parsley, organic black pepper, organic natural flavors (contain corn and dairy derivatives), lactic acid.

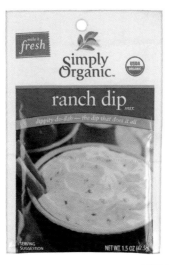

Savvy Pick

Using MSG in its dip is a surefire way for Hidden Valley to make a tasty, hard-to-stop-eating snack. But given that MSG is linked to an increased appetite in lab animals, this is bad news—especially if you are enjoying the dip with chips that are already hard to stop eating after only just a few.

Get Creative

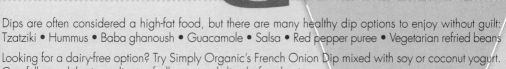

Dips are often considered a high-fat food, but there are many healthy dip options to enjoy without guilt: Tzatziki • Hummus • Baba ghanoush • Guacamole • Salsa • Red pepper puree • Vegetarian refried beans

Looking for a dairy-free option? Try Simply Organic's French Onion Dip mixed with soy or coconut yogurt. Carefully read the ingredients of all prepared dips before buying.

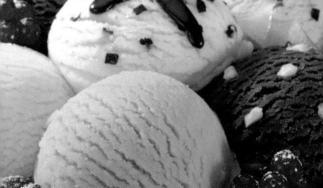

ice cream & other frozen treats

5

GOT MILK?
or NOT milk?

If your body and cow's milk products such as ice cream don't get along, there are some great-tasting dairy-free ice-cream alternatives. Look for products made from coconut milk, rice milk, or soy, which are all lactose free and cholesterol free.

I scream, you scream, we all scream for ice cream.

WHY WE ♥ Frozen Treats

There are few pleasures on earth sweeter than a great big scoop of ice cream on a hot summer day. Ice cream is about as close to a national frozen treat as you can get, with more than 90 percent of American households reporting they consume at least a little bit of ice cream each year.

WORST INGREDIENTS

we found in frozen treats

- Artificial colors
- Artificial flavors
- Artificial sweeteners
- High-fructose corn syrup (HFCS)
- Partially hydrogenated oils (trans fats)
- Polysorbate 65
- Polysorbate 80
- Sodium benzoate

also beware of

- Annatto color
- Caramel color
- Carrageenan
- Margarine (may contain trans fats)
- Potassium sorbate
- Propylene glycol, propylene glycol monostearate
- Sodium carboxymethylcellulose

📖 For definitions of these ingredients, refer to the glossary.

Good News!

Most of the brands of vanilla and chocolate ice cream that we looked at were clean. They were made with basic ingredients such as milk, sugar, cream, and natural flavor. But just to be on the safe side, always read the label before putting the package in your shopping cart.

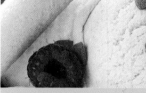

Reasons You Might Be Craving . . . *Ice Cream*

ALLERGY OR INTOLERANCE

It's possible to crave foods that you are allergic to. The most common food allergies and/or intolerances are to dairy, soy, wheat, sugar, peanuts, eggs, and tomatoes.

STRESS

Stress causes a rise in the hormone cortisol and a decrease in serotonin, also known as the body's "feel good" brain chemical. When our serotonin levels get low, we tend to crave foods that will help release serotonin in the brain, like ice cream and other carbohydrates.

YOU CAN'T SLEEP

If you crave a bowl of ice cream before bed, it's probably because your body is searching for ways to produce serotonin, which also helps you sleep soundly. If this is the case, try eating yogurt instead.

savvy fact

Despite what chocoholics might think, the most popular flavor of ice cream in North America is vanilla, followed by chocolate, and then cookies and cream.

Food *for* Thought

Serotonin, the Anti-stress, "Feel Good" Brain Chemical

There's a reason why so many people keep a bucket of double fudge chocolate ice cream in the freezer for when they absolutely must have their "comfort food." These foods produce serotonin, which makes us feel better and helps regulate the sleep cycle (circadian rhythm). Produced by the amino acid L-tryptophan, serotonin is found in dairy products such as ice cream, yogurt, and milk, as well as in turkey, bread, pasta, rice, potatoes, and cereal. Low serotonin levels lead to:

Overeating ("the munchies") • Insomnia
Restlessness • Depression • Anxiety • Carb cravings

Instead of eating a bowl of ice cream, these nutrients (in food and supplements) support a good mood: B vitamins, magnesium, and omega-3.

Brain FREEEEZZZZE

Gobbled down too much of a **frozen treat** too fast? The technical term for the cold-induced headache known as brain freeze is sphenopalatine ganglioneuralgia. Brain freeze results when something cold touches the roof of the mouth. Luckily there's a simple way to prevent brain freeze: **slow down!** If you already feel that cold ache creeping up your brain stem, press your tongue against the roof of your mouth to warm the area. Warning: you may be more susceptible to brain freeze if you're prone to migraines.

DON'T Be Misled

Many low-fat / low-carb ice creams are full of chemicals including artificial sweeteners. High-quality ice cream, although not low in calories and fat, is made from all-natural ingredients such as milk, cream, and sugar. So, pick your poison: calories or chemicals.

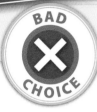

french vanilla ice cream

Edy's Ice Cream
Rich & Creamy Grand—French Vanilla

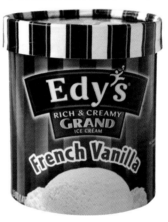

Yellow 5 and Yellow 6
These petroleum-based dyes are used to color foods, cosmetics, and other products. Yellow 5, Tartrazine, may cause hyperactivity in children, allergies, asthma, and other health issues. Yellow 6, Sunset Yellow, has been shown to cause tumors in animals, stomach cramps, and rashes, and may cause hyperactivity in children.

Carrageenan
This thickening agent is often used to replace gelatin, which is usually made from animal products. While more research on this ingredient is needed, new evidence indicates that it could be a factor in intestinal disease in humans.

Dextrose
A sugar and corn derivative, dextrose is added to many foods as a sweetener. In fact, the average person consumes about 25 pounds of dextrose a year.

Nutrition Facts
Serving size ½ cup

Calories 150	Calories from fat 80
Total fat 9 g	
Saturated fat 5 g	
Trans fat 0 g	
Cholesterol 50 mg	
Sodium 35 mg	
Total carbohydrates 16 g	
Dietary fiber 0 g	
Sugars 11 g	
Protein 2 g	

INGREDIENTS: milk, cream, skim milk, corn syrup, sugar, egg yolks, natural flavor, cellulose gum, monoglycerides and diglycerides, ground vanilla beans, guar gum, carrageenan, Yellow 5, Yellow 6, dextrose.

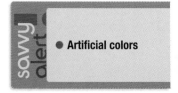

savvy alert

● Artificial colors

D-I-Y
banana ice treats
For a healthy and delicious all-natural frozen treat, freeze ripe bananas, blend in a food processor, and then refreeze them to make "banana ice cream." Add real vanilla extract for flavor.

365 Ice Cream (Whole Foods Market Brand)
French Vanilla

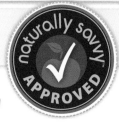

Nutrition Facts
Serving size ½ cup (68 g)

Calories 150	Calories from fat 80
Total fat 8 g	
Saturated fat 5 g	
Trans fat 0 g	
Cholesterol 55 mg	
Sodium 45 mg	
Total carbohydrates 15 g	
Dietary fiber 0 g	
Sugars 15 g	
Protein 3 g	

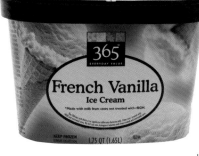

INGREDIENTS: milk, cream, sugar, condensed skim milk, custard base (frozen sugar, egg yolks [egg yolks, sugar], water, evaporated milk, sweetened condensed milk, invert sugar, butter [cream and salt], fructose, brown sugar, natural flavors, salt, annatto, locust bean gum, guar gum, vanilla bean seeds, vanilla extract (water, ethyl alcohol, natural flavor), annatto extract (color).

Savvy Pick
While Edy's ice cream contains artificial dyes, Whole Foods Market's in-house brand, 365, is made with milk free of rBGH (recombinant bovine growth hormone)—a genetically engineered hormone given to cows to increase their milk supply. Since both products have about the same amount of fat and calories per serving, our Savvy opinion is that Whole Foods 365 French Vanilla Ice Cream is definitely the way to go.

Honorable Mention
❖ Three Twins *Madagascar Vanilla*

Crazy for Coconut

If you suffer from lactose intolerance, a dairy allergy, or you're vegan, you'll love the dairy-free option: **Purely Decadent's Vanilla Bean Non-Dairy Frozen Dessert**. Made with creamy vanilla coconut milk, it's a delicious, non-dairy substitute for vanilla ice cream.

cookie dough ice cream

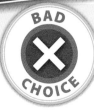

BAD ✗ **CHOICE**

Blue Bunny Premium Ice Cream
Super Chunky Cookie Dough

Partially hydrogenated oils *trans fats*
Trans fats raise your bad (LDL) cholesterol levels and lower your good (HDL) cholesterol levels.

Margarine
The word margarine on ingredient labels usually indicates that the product contains trans fat—unless "non-hydrogenated" margarine is specified on the label.

Gluten
Most cookie dough ice creams contain gluten since it is in the cookie dough.

Nutrition Facts

Serving size ½ cup

Calories 180	Calories from fat 80
Total fat 9 g	
Saturated fat 5 g	
Trans fat 0 g	
Cholesterol 25 mg	
Sodium 110 mg	
Total carbohydrates 24 g	
Dietary fiber 0 g	
Sugars 21 g	
Protein 3 g	

savvy alert

- **Partially hydrogenated oils** *trans fats*
- **Sodium benzoate** *preservative*
- **Artificial flavor**
- **Margarine** *may contain trans fats*

INGREDIENTS: milk, cream, sugar, cookie dough chunks (brown sugar, wheat flour, margarine [partially hydrogenated soybean and cottonseed oils, water, salt, monoglycerides, soy lecithin, sodium benzoate (preservative), artificial flavor, beta-carotene, vitamin A palmitate], sugar, chocolate [sugar, chocolate liquor, cocoa butter, dextrose, soy lecithin], water, natural flavor, food starch, baking soda, salt, soy lecithin), revel (sugar, corn syrup, brown sugar, corn oil, wheat flour, water, butter, nonfat milk, salt, natural flavor, soy lecithin), buttermilk, flavor base (brown sugar, water, molasses, flour, salt, sodium benzoate and potassium sorbate [preservative]), chocolate flakes (sugar, chocolate liquor, cocoa butter, soy lecithin, vanilla extract, salt), corn syrup, carob bean gum, guar gum, monoglycerides and diglycerides, carrageenan.

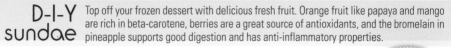

D-I-Y sundae Top off your frozen dessert with delicious fresh fruit. Orange fruit like papaya and mango are rich in beta-carotene, berries are a great source of antioxidants, and the bromelain in pineapple supports good digestion and has anti-inflammatory properties.

Breyers All Natural Ice Cream
Chocolate Chip Cookie Dough

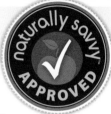

Nutrition Facts
Serving size ½ cup

Calories 160	Calories from fat 70
Total fat 8 g	
Saturated fat 5 g	
Trans fat 0 g	
Cholesterol 15 mg	
Sodium 50 mg	
Total carbohydrates 20 g	
Dietary fiber 0 g	
Sugars 17 g	
Protein 2 g	

INGREDIENTS: ice cream: milk, cream, sugar, whey, natural flavor, natural tara gum; chocolate chip cookie dough pieces: wheat flour, sugar, brown sugar, palm oil, water, soybean oil, chocolate liquor, salt, cocoa butter, cornstarch, natural flavor, soy lecithin, baking soda; chocolate flavored chips: sugar, coconut oil, cocoa (processed with alkali), milk fat, soy lecithin, natural flavor.

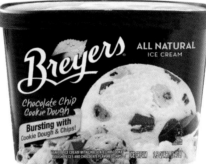

Savvy Pick
With no trans fats, no artificial flavors, half the sodium, fewer calories, and less fat than Blue Bunny, Breyers is our top pick for cookie dough ice cream. Dig in!

Honorable Mentions
❖ Ben & Jerry's
Chocolate Chip Cookie Dough

❖ Purely Decadent (gluten free)
Coconut Milk Non-Dairy Frozen Dessert—Cookie Dough

savvy serving

The average serving size for ice cream is half a cup. That's about the size of a tennis ball. If your preference is a double-scoop waffle cone, chances are you're getting too much of a good thing.

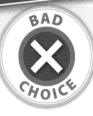

mint chocolate chip ice cream

Edy's Ice Cream
Rich & Creamy Grand—Mint Chocolate Chip

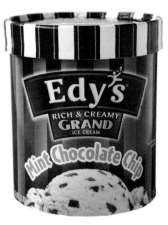

Nutrition Facts
Serving size ½ cup

Calories 150	Calories from fat 70

Total fat 8 g
Saturated fat 6 g
Trans fat 0 g
Cholesterol 20 mg
Sodium 35 mg
Total carbohydrates 18 g
Dietary fiber 0 g
Sugars 16 g
Protein 2 g

INGREDIENTS: skim milk, cream, sugar, chocolaty chips (sugar, coconut oil, cocoa processed with alkali (dutched cocoa), fractionated palm kernel oil, cocoa, soy lecithin, salt, natural flavor), corn syrup, whey, molasses, natural flavor, acacia gum, guar gum, Yellow 5, Blue 1, carob bean gum, carrageenan, xanthan gum.

Don't be misled
Most conventional brands of mint ice creams get their minty green shade from artificial colors. Mint ice creams don't have to be green, and the greener they are, the more artificial color you may be eating.

Artificial color
According to the FDA, "*Without color additives, colas wouldn't be brown, margarine wouldn't be yellow, and mint ice cream wouldn't be green. Color additives are now recognized as an important part of practically all processed foods we eat.*" We are optimistic that one day this won't be the case.

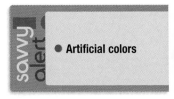

savvy alert

● Artificial colors

Turkey Hill—All Natural Ice Cream
Philadelphia Style—Mint Chocolate Chip

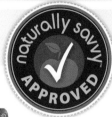

Nutrition Facts
Serving size ½ cup (69 g)

Calories 160	Calories from fat 80
Total fat 9 g	
Saturated fat 5 g	
Trans fat 0 g	
Cholesterol 25 mg	
Sodium 45 mg	
Total carbohydrates 18 g	
Dietary fiber 0 g	
Sugars 18 g	
Protein 3 g	

INGREDIENTS: cream, nonfat milk, sugar, chocolate chips (sugar, chocolate liquor, cocoa butter, lecithin, vanilla), oil of peppermint.

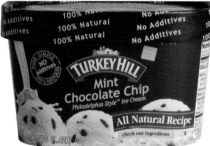

Savvy Pick

Turkey Hill Choco Mint Chip has no artificial colors, and uses real peppermint for flavor. But not all of its ice cream lines are natural, so be sure to look for "All Natural Recipe" on the package.

Honorable Mention

❖ Purely Decadent
*Coconut Milk Frozen Dessert
Mint Chip*

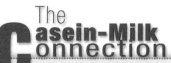

The Casein-Milk Connection

asein is one of the most common allergenic proteins in cow's milk. The word "non-dairy" does not necessarily mean that a product doesn't contain casein, and many non-dairy products on the market (including soy cheese, almond cheese, and rice cheese) use casein as a primary protein-boosting ingredient. On a food label, casein may be listed as caseinate, calcium caseinate, ammonium caseinate, magnesium caseinate, potassium caseinate, and sodium caseinate.

low-fat ice cream—cookies n' cream

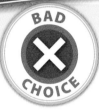

BAD ✗ CHOICE

Skinny Cow Low-Fat Ice Cream
Cookies 'N Cream

Low-fat does not always mean healthy

Many low-fat frozen desserts (including this one) give the impression they are healthy, but if that's the case, they should not have unhealthy partially hydrogenated oil (trans fats) and high-fructose corn syrup in them. Not to mention the fact that high-fructose corn syrup contributes to weight gain.

What is polydextrose?

Polydextrose is a mixture of dextrose (corn sugar) and sorbitol. The FDA requires that all products containing more than 15 grams of polydextrose to put a warning on the label: "*Sensitive individuals may experience a laxative effect from excessive consumption of this product.*"

Nutrition Facts

Serving size 1 container
(5.8 fl oz = 0.725 cups)

Calories 150	Calories from fat 20

Total fat 2 g	
Saturated fat 1 g	
Trans fat 0 g	
Cholesterol 5 mg	
Sodium 90 mg	
Total carbohydrates 29 g	
Dietary fiber 4 g	
Sugars 18 g	
Protein 5 g	

INGREDIENTS: skim milk, sugar, corn syrup, cookie crumbs (bleached wheat flour, sugar, vegetable shortening [partially hydrogenated soybean oil, partially hydrogenated cottonseed oil], cocoa processed with alkali, high-fructose corn syrup, caramel color, chocolate, leavening [baking soda, ammonium bicarbonate], salt, cornstarch, whey, soy lecithin), polydextrose, whey protein, cream, calcium carbonate, inulin (dietary fiber), propylene glycol monostearate, microcrystalline cellulose, sodium carboxymethylcellulose, guar gum, monoglycerides, sorbitol, carob bean gum, citric acid, vitamin A palmitate, carrageenan, natural flavor, salt.

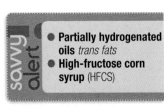

savvy alert

- **Partially hydrogenated oils** *trans fats*
- **High-fructose corn syrup** (HFCS)

goat milk ice cream

Creamy and delicious, goat's milk products can be less allergenic and more easily digested than cow's milk products. If you're allergic to dairy products, experiment with goat's milk ice cream. A brand we like is Laloos.

Breyers Smooth & Dreamy ½ Fat
Cookies & Cream

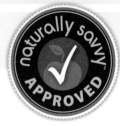

Nutrition Facts
Serving size ½ cup (67 g)

Calories 130	Calories from fat 35
Total fat 4 g	
Saturated fat 2.5 g	
Trans fat 0 g	
Cholesterol 20 mg	
Sodium 95 mg	
Total carbohydrates 21 g	
Dietary fiber 0 g	
Sugars 17 g	
Protein 3 g	

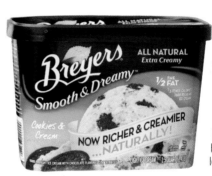

INGREDIENTS: ice cream: skim milk, sugar, corn syrup, cream, whey, egg yolk portions, carob bean gum, salt, natural flavor, beta-carotene (Vitamin A); cookies: sugar, wheat flour, palm and palm kernel oil, cocoa processed with alkali, salt, sodium bicarbonate, soy lecithin, natural flavor.

Savvy Pick
When it comes to quality, Breyers ½ Fat Cookies & Cream runs circles around Skinny Cow. So moove over, Skinny Cow! Breyers Smooth & Dreamy ½ Fat Cookies & Cream is our low-fat pick.

THE SKINNY ON FAT

There's no denying it: real ice cream is high in fat. However, low-fat products are typically made by adding carbs (sugar) and/or fillers (emulsifiers and thickeners) to replace the fat; but carbs that aren't "burned" by physical activity are turned into fat by your body—so although low-fat ice cream has less fat per serving, in the end your body will store it the same way. You're better off with a serving of real, full-fat ice cream and getting more exercise.

frozen yogurt—strawberry

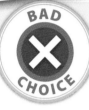

Hood
Frozen Yogurt—Fat Free—Strawberry

Artificial color

In our own households we've noticed that when our kids eat snacks or foods laden with artificial colors, their behavior is affected within only ten minutes (we call it "the crazies"). If you notice that your child's conduct changes after eating a certain food, take note—it could be the result of an additive.

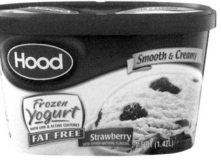

A closer look at the label

Hood is riding the popular and trendy probiotic train, advertising that its fat-free frozen yogurts contain live and active cultures and are free of fat and cholesterol. Although a look at the ingredients reveals artificial colors (including Blue 1 and the dangerous Red 40), don't be fooled, probiotics won't offset the harm.

Made with natural flavors

This statement appears on the front of the package, and while it is true, it doesn't mean this frozen yogurt is made *only* with natural flavors. There is artificial stuff in there too.

Nutrition Facts
Serving size ½ cup (65 g)

Calices (80)	Calories from fat 0
Total fat (0 g)	
Saturated fat 0 g	
Trans fat (0 g)	
Cholesterol 0 mg	
Sodium (45 mg)	
Total carbohydrates 18 g	
Dietary fiber 0 g	
Sugars 12 g	
Protein 3 g	

INGREDIENTS: nonfat milk, cultured non-fat milk, sugar, strawberries, corn syrup, maltodextrin, natural flavors, modified cornstarch, monoglycerides and diglycerides, locust bean gum, cellulose gum, guar gum, citric acid, carrageenan, Red 40, Blue 1. Contains live and active cultures, including L. acidophilus and bifidobacterium.

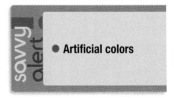

• Artificial colors

savvy
serving

The average serving size for fro-yo is the same as ice cream—a half cup. But just because this treat is made from yogurt, it doesn't give you permission to overindulge. Measure your portions so that you know exactly how much you are eating.

Stonyfield Organic
Strawberry-licious Nonfat Frozen Yogurt

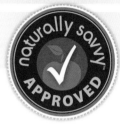

Nutrition Facts
Serving size ½ cup (100 g)

Calories 100	Calories from fat 0
Total fat 0 g	
Saturated fat 0 g	
Trans fat 0 g	
Cholesterol Less than 5 mg	
Sodium 55 mg	
Total carbohydrates 21 g	
Dietary fiber 0 g	
Sugars 19 g	
Protein 4 g	

INGREDIENTS: cultured, pasteurized, organic nonfat milk, naturally milled organic sugar, organic strawberry puree, organic strawberries, organic rice syrup, organic flavor, whey protein concentrate, pectin, organic locust bean gum, organic guar gum, natural flavor, organic beet, organic carrot, organic black currant juice concentrates (color). Contains: s. thermophilus, l. bulgaricus, l. acidophilus, bifidus, and l. casei live active cultures.

Savvy Pick
In a Stonyfield Farm half-cup serving, you get 100 grams of organic goodness versus 65 grams from Hood—so you get more quality bang for your buck. Added bonus: Stonyfield Farm's fat-free frozen yogurt is certified organic and derived from natural ingredients such as fruit, fruit juice, vegetable juice, and plants.

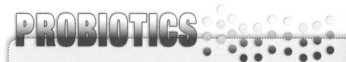

Probiotic foods and supplements contain the beneficial bacterial cultures that help the body's naturally occurring intestinal flora re-establish itself. Hundreds of bacterial strains inhabit the human colon. The most important varieties are Lactobacillus acidophilus and Bifidobacterium bifidus. The best known example of a probiotic food is organic plain yogurt, but other fermented foods containing similar bacteria include miso (as in miso soup), sauerkraut, and kefir. Include these foods in your diet regularly.

sherbet—raspberry

BAD
X
CHOICE

Perry's Ice Cream
Raspberry Sherbet

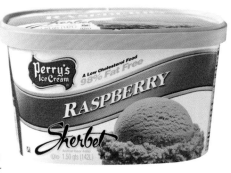

What is malic acid?
Extracted from apples, it adds a tart flavor to food and is an important nutrient. In fact, it may be helpful for those with fibromyalgia. Speak to your health care practitioner for more information.

High-fructose corn syrup
The worst kind of sugar, HFCS is a major contributor to weight gain. Foods with fructose fail to "turn off" your hunger signals, so you're still hungry even after eating (or drinking) your snack. According to one research study, HFCS does not stimulate leptin, the hormone that tells you that you're full, but rather increases levels of ghrelin, the hormone that tells you you're still hungry.

Nutrition Facts
Serving size ½ cup (87 g)

Calories 120	Calories from fat 10
Total fat 1.5 g	
Saturated fat 1 g	
Trans fat 0 g	
Cholesterol 5 mg	
Sodium 20 mg	
Total carbohydrates 27 g	
Dietary fiber 0 g	
Sugars 25 g	
Protein 1 g	

Ingredients: milk, liquid sugar, water, corn syrup, raspberry puree (concentrated grape juice, raspberry puree, concentrated raspberry juice, high-fructose corn syrup, malic acid, water, natural flavors), citric acid, skim milk, buttermilk, natural and artificial raspberry flavor, methyl cellulose, guar gum, monoglycerides and diglycerides, locust bean gum, dextrose, Red 40.

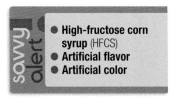

savvy alert
- **High-fructose corn syrup** (HFCS)
- **Artificial flavor**
- **Artificial color**

sherbet vs sorbet

Sherbet is made from 1 to 2 percent milk fat and is sweeter than ice cream. Sorbet is made from a fruit puree or juice and contains no dairy products.

GaGa's SherBetter
Raspberry Pint

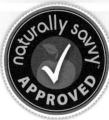

naturally savvy APPROVED

Nutrition Facts

Serving size ½ cup (99 g)

Calories 150	Calories from fat 35

Total fat 3.5 g
Saturated fat 2.5 g
Trans fat 0 g
Cholesterol 15 mg
Sodium 30 mg
Total carbohydrates 28 g
Dietary fiber 0 g
Sugars 28 g
Protein 2 g

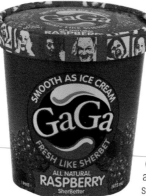

Savvy Pick
We went gaga over GaGa's creamy SherBetter sherbet because it is made with only one type of sugar as opposed to Perry's four sugars, which include high-fructose corn syrup.

Ingredients: milk, liquid cane sugar, cream, skim milk, red raspberry puree (red raspberries, red raspberry concentrate, water), citric acid, ascorbic acid, guar gum, xanthan gum.

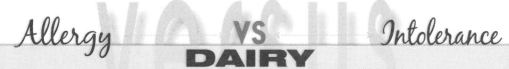

Allergy **VS** *Intolerance*
DAIRY

An allergy is our body's overreaction to something that is not normally harmful, like milk or peanuts. When the body identifies something as foreign, the immune system responds by producing inflammation somewhere in the body, like the skin or respiratory system. A dairy intolerance, on the other hand, such as lactose intolerance, affects only the digestive system.

ice cream sandwiches

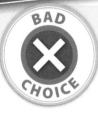

BAD ✗ CHOICE

Klondike
Classic Vanilla Sandwiches

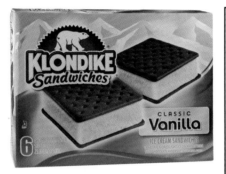

Corn allergies
High-fructose corn syrup, corn syrup, and modified cornstarch in one ice-cream bar. This product is a no-no for anyone with corn allergies.

Nutrition Facts
Serving size 1 sandwich (73 g)

Calories 180	Calories from fat 40
Total fat 4.5 g	
Saturated fat 2.5 g	
Trans fat 0 g	
Cholesterol 10 mg	
Sodium 150 mg	
Total carbohydrates 31 g	
Dietary fiber Less than 1 g	
Sugars 16 g	
Protein 3 g	

Corn syrup vs high-fructose corn syrup (HFCS)
Corn syrup and high-fructose corn syrup are very different sweeteners. Corn syrup is created by heating cornstarch to temperatures high enough to break it down into glucose (sugar). Sometimes this sugar isn't sweet enough for food producers, so to convert it to high-fructose corn syrup, it goes through additional processing to change some of the molecules into fructose, a sweeter and far more unhealthy compound.

INGREDIENTS: light ice cream: nonfat milk, sugar, corn syrup, milk fat, whey, maltodextrin, propylene glycol monoesters, cellulose gel, monoglycerides and diglycerides, cellulose gum, locust bean gum, guar gum, polysorbate 80, carrageenan, natural and artificial flavors, caramel color, annatto (color), vitamin A palmitate; wafer: bleached wheat flour, sugar, palm oil, caramel color, dextrose, high-fructose corn syrup, modified cornstarch, baking soda, salt, cocoa, soy lecithin.

Food additives that may contain corn
Many food additives are derived from corn, including maltodextrin, polydextrose, polysorbates, and propylene glycol monostearate.

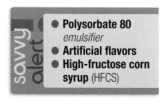

savvy alert

- **Polysorbate 80** *emulsifier*
- **Artificial flavors**
- **High-fructose corn syrup** (HFCS)

good news for gluten free

If you avoid gluten but crave ice cream sandwiches, Julie's Organic Ice Cream makes a gluten-free variety.

Julie's Organic
Vanilla Ice Cream Sandwiches

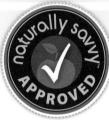

Nutrition Facts

Serving size 1 sandwich (80 g)

Calories 160	Calories from fat 70
Total fat 8 g	
Saturated fat 4.5 g	
Trans fat 0 g	
Cholesterol 35 mg	
Sodium 105 mg	
Total carbohydrates 18 g	
Dietary fiber 0 g	
Sugars 9 g	
Protein 3 g	

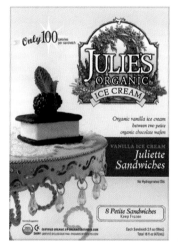

INGREDIENTS: ice cream: fresh organic cream, organic dehydrated cane juice, organic skim milk, organic egg yolks, organic vanilla, carob bean gum, guar gum; **chocolate wafer:** organic unenriched flour, organic dehydrated cane juice, water, organic palm oil, caramel color, organic soy flour, baking soda, soy lecithin, salt, organic vanilla, organic cocoa.

Savvy Pick

What would we do for a Klondike Bar? Considering its ingredients—nothing. Julie's ice cream sandwiches have more fat and calories, but less sugar and sodium. Big plus: they are also organic, so they don't contain any pesticides, hormones, or other chemical additives.

Honorable Mentions

⚜ Tofutti Vanilla Cuties *(soy)*

⚜ So Delicious
  Vanilla Minis Sandwich (coconut)

savvyFACT

A Danish study found that organic milk from grass-fed cows contained about 50 percent more vitamin E and more omega-3 fats—which combat inflammation and heart disease—than conventionally produced milk. The organic milk also had more antioxidants, including 142 percent more beta-carotene.

fudge bars

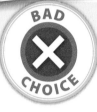

Fudgsicle
Original Fudge Bars

Polysorbate 80
This emulsifier is used in products such as ice cream to keep the ingredients mixed, which helps maintain the product's texture and shape. The Environmental Working Group (EWG) reports that polysorbate 80 is linked to cancer as well as nervous system and reproductive toxicity. Furthermore, studies have shown it can cause severe allergic reactions. It's also used in personal care products such as creams and lotions, so read labels carefully and shop around.

Corn syrup
Although it's not as bad as high-fructose corn syrup, this sweetener, made from corn, is still highly refined and will send your blood sugar soaring. It's in both conventional and natural products.

Chocolate processed with alkali
Dutch processing—adding alkali to chocolate to produce a smoother taste and texture—can damage up to 90 percent of the antioxidants in cacao. Luckily, chocolate is so rich in antioxidants that even after processing it still contains antioxidants.

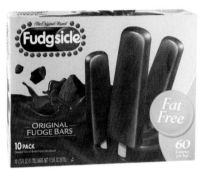

Nutrition Facts
Serving size 1 bar (65 g)

Calories 60	Calories from fat 15
Total fat 1.5 g	
Saturated fat 1 g	
Trans fat 0 g	
Cholesterol 0 mg	
Sodium 55 mg	
Total carbohydrates 12 g	
Dietary fiber 1 g	
Sugars 9 g	
Protein 1 g	

INGREDIENTS: nonfat milk, sugar, corn syrup, whey, high-fructose corn syrup, water, palm oil, cocoa processed with alkali, tricalcium phosphate, monoglycerides and diglycerides, cellulose gum, guar gum, malt powder, salt, polysorbate 80, polysorbate 65, carrageenan.

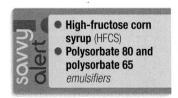

savvy alert

- **High-fructose corn syrup** (HFCS)
- **Polysorbate 80 and polysorbate 65** *emulsifiers*

portion control

The calories, fat, and sodium listed on a product might seem acceptable, but sometimes the serving size is pretty small. Remember: if you double the portion, you double the number of calories, fat, and sodium per serving.

Jala
Chocolate Fudge Ice Cream Bars

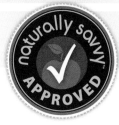

Nutrition Facts

Serving size 1 bar (76 g)

Calories 110	Calories from fat 10
Total fat 1 g	
Saturated fat 0 g	
Trans fat 0 g	
Cholesterol 5 mg	
Sodium 70 mg	
Total carbohydrates 24 g	
Dietary fiber Less than 1 gram	
Sugars 17 g	
Protein 4 g	

Ingredients: skim milk, whole milk, sugar, corn syrup, whey, cocoa processed with alkali, nonfat dry milk, maltodextrin, dextrose, soy lecithin, guar gum, xanthan gum, carrageenan, Lactobacillus acidophilus, Bifidobacterium lactis, vitamin A palmitate.

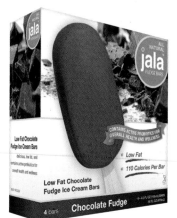

Savvy Pick

Fudgsicle's frozen fudge bars contain numerous red flags including high-fructose corn syrup and polysorbates. Jala bars are super light and creamy. It's our Savvy Pick—bar none!

Honorable Mentions

‡ Sweet Nothings
  Non-Dairy Fudge Bars

‡ So Delicious
  Fudge Bars

‡ FrütStix's
  FudgStix Lite

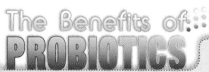

The Benefits of PROBIOTICS

Science is proving the benefits of a diet rich in probiotics—which include boosting immunity, improving digestion, and promoting intestinal health (including preventing constipation). If probiotics aren't included in your diet daily, supplements are available. When you're buying probiotics, the minimum dose you should take is one billion colony forming units, or cfu. For theraputic use, look for a product with ten billion cfu. We like Bio-K+ and Natren because both brands have been well researched and scientifically documented.

fruit-flavored ice bars

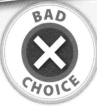

Popsicle
Rainbow

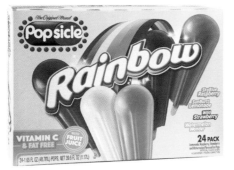

 Misleading marketing

The front of the Popsicle box reads, "Vitamin C & Fat Free, with Fruit Juice," giving the impression this is a healthy product. Unfortunately this isn't the case when you turn the box over to read the ingredients. Start paying attention to packaging when you're shopping. You'll find that the front of the box will often boast which additives the product does not have (such as artificial flavors and certain preservatives). However, when you look at the ingredients list, you'll find which additives they left out on purpose to mislead you into thinking the product is healthier than it really is.

 High-fructose corn syrup

Gram for gram, HFCS has nearly the same number of calories as table sugar (sucrose), but the health implications of eating HFCS are far worse. There is growing evidence that excess fructose—as in high-fructose corn syrup—may promote insulin resistance and eventually type 2 diabetes.

Nutrition Facts
Serving size 1 bar (53 g)

Calories 45	Calories from fat 0

Total fat 0 g	
Saturated fat 0 g	
Trans fat 0 g	
Cholesterol 0 mg	
Sodium 0 mg	
Total carbohydrates 11 g	
Dietary fiber 0 g	
Sugars 8 g	
Protein 0 g	

INGREDIENTS: water, pear juice from concentrate, liquid sugar (sugar, water), high-fructose corn syrup, corn syrup, lemon juice from concentrate, strawberry juice from concentrate, raspberry juice from concentrate, watermelon juice from concentrate, citric acid, malic acid, guar gum, natural and artificial flavors, locust bean gum, ascorbic acid, Yellow 5, Red 40, Blue 1.

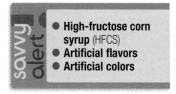

savvy alert
- **High-fructose corn syrup** (HFCS)
- **Artificial flavors**
- **Artificial colors**

D-I-Y fruit bars

The deeper the color of a juice or fruit, the more antioxidants it has. Make your own fruit bars with healthy juices, such as cranberry, blueberry, acai, pomegranate, and mango. Blend the ingredients until smooth, pour into a BPA-free ice pop mold, and freeze.

Breyers
Pure Fruit Bars

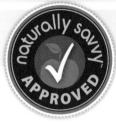

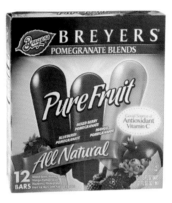

Nutrition Facts

Serving size 1 bar (1.75 fl oz)

Calories 40	Calories from fat 0
Total fat 0 g	
Saturated fat 0 g	
Trans fat 0 g	
Cholesterol 0 mg	
Sodium 0 mg	
Total carbohydrates 10 g	
Dietary fiber 0 g	
Sugars 9 g	
Protein 0 g	

Savvy Pick

Breyers Pure Fruit Bars avoid artificial coloring, so they get our vote. Rainbow Popsicles are made with an array of healthy juices—lemon, strawberry, raspberry, and watermelon—it's a shame to taint them with artificial colors and high-fructose corn syrup.

INGREDIENTS: strawberry: water, fructose, strawberries and strawberry puree, apple puree concentrate, beet juice concentrate (color), acerola cherry concentrate, pectin, guar gum, locust bean gum, citric acid, natural flavor, turmeric (color); raspberry: water, fructose, raspberry puree, apple puree concentrate, natural flavor, beet juice concentrate (color), acerola cherry concentrate, pectin, guar gum, locust bean gum, citric acid; orange: water, orange juice concentrate, fructose, orange.

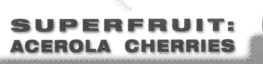

SUPERFRUIT: ACEROLA CHERRIES

Providing far more nutrients than most other fruits, acerola cherries are one of our favorites. They pack significant amounts of vitamin A, folate, potassium, and vitamin C (about 800 milligrams in a quarter cup!). They also contain a phytonutrient called anthocyanin, which has anti-inflammatory properties and performs similarly to over-the-counter painkillers.

freezer pops

Fla-Vor-Ice
Fruity Flavors

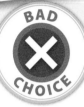

Artificial colors
A large concern about the usage of artificial colors stems from the many ingredients used to make them. According to the Center for Science in the Public Interest (CSPI), artificial colors are made with contaminants that are known carcinogens.

High-fructose corn syrup (HFCS)
The USDA calculates that the average American consumes 35.7 pounds of HFCS per year. This doesn't even include all the other sweeteners in our diet.

High-fructose corn syrup (HFCS)
The corn used to make high-fructose corn syrup is not the same corn that we eat. It is a specific type of corn called yellow dent corn, most of which is grown in Iowa.

Nutrition Facts
Serving size 43 g

Calories 25	Calories from fat 0
Total fat 0 g	
Saturated fat 0 g	
Trans fat 0 g	
Cholesterol 0 mg	
Sodium 0 mg	
Total carbohydrates 6 g	
Dietary fiber 0 g	
Sugars 6 g	
Protein 0 g	

INGREDIENTS: water, high-fructose corn syrup, fruit juice (contains one or more of the following: apple, grape, and/or pear juice from concentrate). Contains less than 2 percent each of citric acid and/or fumaric acid, natural and artificial flavors, sodium benzoate and potassium sorbate (preservatives), Red 40, Yellow 5, Yellow 6, Blue 1.

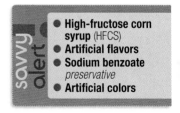

savvy alert
- **High-fructose corn syrup** (HFCS)
- **Artificial flavors**
- **Sodium benzoate** *preservative*
- **Artificial colors**

freezie-fun Your kids will love making their own freezies. Think outside the box— make them with herbal tea, chocolate milk, pink lemonade and even water.

Cool Fruits
Fruit Juice Freezers—Grape & Cherry

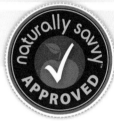

Nutrition Facts
Serving size 3 pops (84 g; 28 g per pop)

Calories 70 (23 per pop) Calories from fat 0	
Total fat 0 g	
Saturated fat 0 g	
Trans fat 0 g	
Cholesterol 0 mg	
Sodium 0 mg	
Total carbohydrates 18 g (6 g per pop)	
Dietary fiber 0 g	
Sugars 18 g (6 g per pop)	
Protein 0 g	

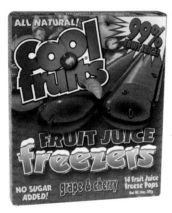

INGREDIENTS: Grape: water, grape and/or pear juice from concentrate, natural color, natural flavor, ascorbic acid (vitamin C), vegetable gum. Cherry: water, grape and/or pear juice from concentrate, lemon juice concentrate, natural color, natural cherry flavor, ascorbic acid (vitamin C), vegetable gum.

Savvy Pick
Freezies are a fantastic treat at kids' events so why not opt for a brand that avoids the artificial colors and HFCS? Cool Fruits freezer pops are made with natural juices. We think they're pretty, well, cool.

Honorable Mention

❖ Power of Fruit
  Frozen Fruit Bars

Check The Serving Size

At first glance, it may look like Cool Fruits has more calories and sugar than Fla-Vor-Ice, but that is because its serving size is for three pops, not one. However, when you break it down, freezer pop for freezer pop, both products have the almost the same amount of calories and fat. This is a great example of why it is important to look at serving sizes carefully before eating a product.

toppings

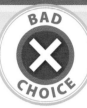

Nestlé Nesquik
Chocolate Syrup

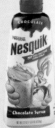

INGREDIENTS: sugar, water, cocoa processed with alkali. Less than 2 percent each of salt, citric acid, artificial flavor, potassium sorbate, xanthan gum, caramel color, Red 40, Blue 1, Yellow 6.

Nutrition Facts
Serving size 1 tbsp (20 g)

Calories	50
Sodium	30 mg
Total carbohydrates	13 g
Sugars 12	

Kraft Jet-Puffed
Marshmallow Creme

INGREDIENTS: corn syrup, sugar, water, egg whites, artificial flavor, cream of tartar, xanthan gum, artificial color (Blue 1).

Nutrition Facts
Serving size 2 tbsp (13 g)

Calories	40
Sodium	10 mg
Total carbohydrates	11 g
Sugars 9 g	

Betty Crocker
Parlor Perfect
Confetti Sprinkles

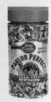

INGREDIENTS: sugar, partially hydrogenated vegetable oil (soybean and cottonseed oil), cornstarch, cocoa processed with alkali, dextrin, carnauba wax, confectioner's glaze, soy lecithin, natural and artificial flavors, Red 40 lake, Yellow 6 lake, Yellow 5 lake, Blue 1 lake, Red 3.

Nutrition Facts
Serving size 1 tsp (4 g)

Calories	20
Total fat	1 g
Total carbohydrates	3 g
Sugars 2 g	

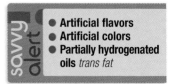

savvy alert
- Artificial flavors
- Artificial colors
- Partially hydrogenated oils *trans* fat

Toppings transform ice cream into a magnificent sundae, but our excitement "bottomed out" when we saw how many artificial ingredients they contained...

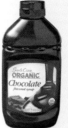

Nutrition Facts
Serving size 2 tbsp (40 g)

Calories 110	(55 per tbsp)
Sodium 15 mg	(7.5 mg per tbsp)
Total carbohydrates 26 g (13 g per tbsp)	
Sugars 24 g (12 g per tbsp)	

INGREDIENTS: organic invert sugar, organic cocoa, organic vanilla extract, salt, xanthan gum.

Santa Cruz Organic
Chocolate
Flavored Syrup

Nutrition Facts
Serving size 2 tbsp (14 g)

Calories 40	
Sodium 5 mg	
Total carbohydrates 9 g	
Sugars 7 g	

INGREDIENTS: brown rice syrup, soy protein, natural flavors, natural gums.

Suzanne's
Ricemellow Crème

Nutrition Facts
Serving size 1 tsp (4 g)

Calories 15	
Total carbohydrates 4 g	
Sugars 3 g	

INGREDIENTS: organic evaporated cane juice, organic corn malt syrup, water, organic natural colors (organic beet powder, organic spinach powder, organic turmeric).

Let's Do . . . Sprinkelz
Natural Dessert Toppings

...Some good detective work led us to these cleaner brands.

cookies

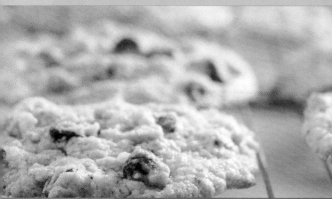

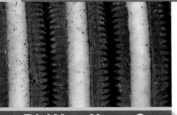

Did You Know?
December 4th
is National Cookie Day!

WHY WE
Cookies

Whether it's a quick pick-me-up during the day or a small after-dinner dessert, just one good cookie can bring big comfort. There's something about these tasty little biscuits that takes us back to our childhood, yet even the most mature of us can enjoy a cookie too. In fact, we love them so much that we consume three hundred cookies per person each year!

Cookies are the perfect portable snack, slipping easily into a purse or brown bag. They make a great after-school snack, go well with coffee or tea, and are easy to bake. And they're a very effective bribe—even for Santa.

WORST INGREDIENTS

we found in **cookies**
+ Artificial colors
+ Artificial flavors
+ Artificial sweeteners
+ High-fructose corn syrup
+ Partially hydrogenated oils (trans fats)
+ Sulfites (sulfur dioxide)
+ TBHQ

also **beware** of
+ Caramel color
+ Hydrogenated oil (may contain trans fats)
+ Sodium stearoyl lactylate

BREAKING THE SUGAR HABIT

If you crave sweets and want to do something about it, try these tips:

- Eat something every three to four hours.

- Add protein to each and every meal and snack.

- Eat foods low on the glycemic index.

- Take probiotics or prebiotics daily.

- Eat carbs with 3 or more grams of fiber per serving.

Reasons You Might Be Craving ... *Cookies*

LOW BLOOD SUGAR

You don't have to be diabetic or hypoglycemic to experience low blood sugar. Cravings for sugar and starch are typically due to a drop in blood glucose (sugar). Signs include intense hunger ("I must eat right now"), a strong desire to eat carbohydrates (especially a sugary food or soda), sudden fatigue, lack of concentration, mood swings, headaches, and nausea up to three hours after eating.

FATIGUE

When your natural energy resources are tapped out, you instinctively look for other ways to perk up. Sugar is the quickest pick-me-up.

CANDIDA

This giant yeast infection thrives on sugar, so you aren't craving carbs—the little critters in your colon are! Speak to your doctor.

For more info about candida, check out www.naturallysavvy.com.

STRESS (or a bad mood)

Stressful situations cause serotonin levels to fall and cortisol levels to rise. When this happens, we naturally crave carbs (cookies, pasta, ice cream . . .) to elevate our mood. But there are better ways to deal with stress than eating cookies. Exercise and deep breathing are good places to start, and look for stress formulas that contain B vitamins at your local natural product store.

> "If I was going to make the world a better place, I would do it with cookies."
>
> —*Maggie Gyllenhaal's character, Ana Pascal, from the movie* Stranger Than Fiction

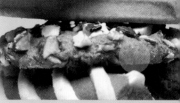

Did You Know?

The Immaculate Baking Co. is credited with baking the largest cookie ever made. Baked in Hendersonville, North Carolina, on May 17, 2003, it was a whopping 102 feet in diameter and weighed in at 38,800 pounds. That's longer than a basketball court and heavier than three Tyrannosaurus rex dinosaurs!

health alert!

To keep blood sugar under control, you need to know how it's behaving. The gold-standard lab test of blood glucose is the hemoglobin A1C test, which measures the average concentration of glucose in the blood over the past few months. An A1C of 5.7 percent to 6.4 percent indicates prediabetes. An A1C of 6.5 percent or above means that you have diabetes. Speak to your doctor for more information.

chocolate chip cookies

BAD CHOICE

Nabisco
Chips Ahoy! Real Chocolate Chip Cookies

Nutrition Facts

Serving size 3 cookies (33 g)

Calories 160	Calories from fat 70
Total fat 8 g	
Saturated fat 2.5 g	
Trans fat 0 g	
Cholesterol 0 mg	
Sodium 110 mg	
Total carbohydrates 22 g	
Dietary fiber 1 g	
Sugars 11 g	
Protein 2 g	

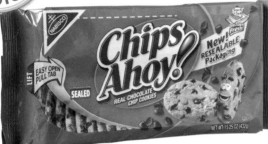

Partially hydrogenated oil
trans fat

The fats we eat are used to make our cell membranes. Since roughly 70 percent of the central nervous system's myelin sheath (the protective covering for the brain's communication neurons and the spinal cord) is composed of fat, when we eat foods containing trans fats, they replace the good fats such as DHA, which are crucial for mental performance. Since this product may contain trans fat, we recommend that you avoid it.

America's favorite cookie

More than 50 percent of the homemade cookies in the United States are chocolate chip.

INGREDIENTS: unbleached enriched flour (wheat flour, niacin, reduced iron, thiamine mononitrate [vitamin B$_1$], riboflavin [vitamin B$_2$], folic acid), semisweet chocolate chips (sugar, chocolate, cocoa butter, dextrose, soy lecithin), sugar, soybean oil and/or partially hydrogenated cottonseed oil, high-fructose corn syrup, leavening (baking soda and/or ammonium phosphate), salt, whey (from milk), natural and artificial flavor, caramel color.

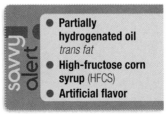

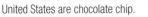

savvy alert
- **Partially hydrogenated oil** *trans fat*
- **High-fructose corn syrup** (HFCS)
- **Artificial flavor**

Burning off the calories of two chocolate chip cookies takes some work:
• 35 minutes of vacuuming • 17 minutes of dancing • 15 minutes of walking briskly
• 13 minutes of swimming, or • 8 minutes of jumping rope.

365 Organic (Whole Foods Market Brand)
Chocolate Chip Cookies

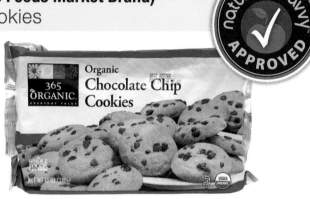

Nutrition Facts
Serving size 2 cookies (30 g)

Calories 150	Calories from fat 60
Total fat 7 g	
Saturated fat 3 g	
Trans fat 0 g	
Cholesterol 0 mg	
Sodium 85 mg	
Total carbohydrates 21 g	
Dietary fiber 1 g	
Sugars 9 g	
Protein 1 g	

INGREDIENTS: organic wheat flour, organic dehydrated cane juice, organic modified palm oil, organic chocolate chips (organic sugar, organic chocolate liquor, organic cocoa butter, organic soy lecithin [emulsifier]), organic invert sugar, sea salt, baking soda, organic vanilla extract, natural flavor, ammonium bicarbonate (leavening).

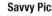

Savvy Pick
We hate to be tough cookies, but Nabisco Chips Ahoy! may contain dangerous trans fats as well as HFCS and artificial flavor. We choose 365.

Honorable Mentions

✛ Lucy's
Chocolate Chip
✛ Glow
Chocolate Chip Cookies (gluten free)

✛ Ian's
Organic Chocolate Chip Cookie Buttons

WEIGHT
CONTROL

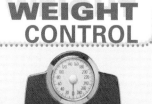

Extra fat isn't gained overnight. It takes 3,500 extra calories (on top of your daily calorie needs) to gain 1 pound of body fat. Sneaking in a treat, such as that last cookie in the package, can add up fast, so take a mental note of what you eat and be picky about where you get your calories. Better yet, keep a food journal and write down everything you put in your mouth. You might be surprised by what you see at the end of the day.

soft chocolate chip cookies

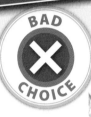

BAD ✗ **CHOICE**

Entenmann's Original Recipe
Chocolate Chip Cookies

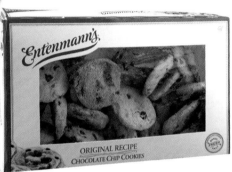

ORIGINAL RECIPE
CHOCOLATE CHIP COOKIES

Nutrition Facts
Serving size 3 cookies (30 g)

Calories 140	Calories from fat 60
Total fat 7 g	
Saturated fat 3 g	
Trans fat 0 g	
Cholesterol Less than 5 mg	
Sodium 80 mg	
Total carbohydrates 20 g	
Dietary fiber Less than 1 g	
Sugars 11 g	
Protein 1 g	

Palm oil
The increasing demand for this oil, which comes from the palm fruit, is leading to deforestation and destruction of the wildlife habitats in Southeast Asia, where the oil is produced. Orangutans, tigers, rhinoceroses, and other endangered wildlife are at risk, and in Malaysia and Indonesia, the world's top producers of palm oil, several species of animals are already critically endangered. Many natural and organic products use palm oil as an ingredient. If you see it on the label of one of your favorite products and you are concerned about its source, contact the company or check out its website to find out if the oil is obtained from environmentally responsible harvesters.

INGREDIENTS: sugar, chocolate chips (sugar, chocolate liquor, cocoa butter, dextrose, chocolate liquor [processed with alkali], soy lecithin, vanillin, vanilla extract), wheat flour, palm oil, bleached wheat flour, high-fructose corn syrup, wheat starch, water, eggs, soybean oil, molasses, modified cornstarch, salt, whey (milk), baking soda, artificial flavor, guar gum, carob bean gum, caramel color, soy protein.

Easy does it
Entenmann's mini cookies might make it easy to grab more than its serving size of three cookies, so you're more likely to overindulge.

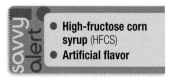

savvy alert
- **High-fructose corn syrup** (HFCS)
- **Artificial flavor**

sugar high

It's estimated that the average American ingests 350 to 475 calories of added sugar every day. Be mindful of the of the various sugar sources in your diet.

Matt's
Real Chocolate Chip Cookies

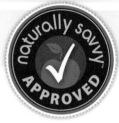

Nutrition Facts

Serving size 1 cookie (30 g)

Calories 139	Calories from fat 62
Total fat 6 g	
Saturated fat 2 g	
Trans fat 0 g	
Cholesterol 23 mg	
Sodium 79 mg	
Total carbohydrates 18.5 g	
Dietary fiber 0.9 g	
Sugars 9.6 g	
Protein 1.5 g	

INGREDIENTS: unbleached wheat flour, real chocolate chips, baking oil (palm, soybean, canola), brown sugar, fresh eggs, sugar, baking soda, salt, vanilla.

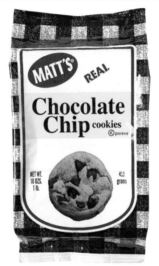

Savvy Pick
Entenmann's cookies contain high-fructose corn syrup and artificial flavor. Matt's mouthwatering soft chocolate chip cookies—made with brown sugar and fresh eggs—taste like they're home baked. Grandma would be proud!

Honorable Mention
❖ Mary's Gone Crackers
   Love Cookies (gluten free)

savvy baking tip

If you love to bake chocolate chip cookies, use baking powder rather than baking soda. Baking soda is much more alkaline and increases the pH of cocoa (as does the Dutch process), significantly decreasing chocolate's antioxidant activity.

sugar-free chocolate chip cookies

BAD X CHOICE

Murray
Sugar-Free Chocolate Chip Cookies

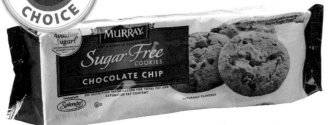

Sugar alcohols
Sugar alcohols such as maltitol and sorbitol are used as a sugar substitute in both conventional and natural products. They are lower in calories and convert to glucose more slowly than sucrose (table sugar). Nonetheless, some diabetics have found that their blood sugar rises if they eat sugar alcohols in large amounts.

Sugar alcohols
They can cause bloating and diarrhea if ingested in large amounts.

Sucralose
Some research suggests that sucralose may cause damage to the kidneys and liver and decreased red blood cell production. The safety of sucralose is still in question. Until further testing, use with caution.

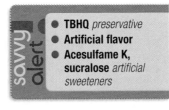

savvy alert
- **TBHQ** *preservative*
- **Artificial flavor**
- **Acesulfame K, sucralose** *artificial sweeteners*

Nutrition Facts
Serving size 3 cookies (32 g)

Calories 150	Calories from fat 80
Total fat 9 g	
Saturated fat 3.5 g	
Trans fat 0 g	
Cholesterol Less than 5 mg	
Sodium 130 mg	
Total carbohydrates 20 g	
Dietary fiber 2 g	
Sugars 0 g	
Protein 2 g	

INGREDIENTS: enriched flour (wheat flour, niacin, reduced iron, thiamine mononitrate [vitamin B$_1$], riboflavin [vitamin B$_2$], folic acid), soybean and palm oil with TBHQ (for freshness), sugar-free chocolate flavored chips (maltitol, chocolate processed with alkali, cocoa butter, soy lecithin, vanilla extract), maltitol, lactitol, polydextrose, maltodextrin, sorbitol.* Contains 2 percent or less of natural and artificial flavor, salt, leavening (baking soda, sodium acid pyrophosphate), eggs, soy lecithin, xanthan gum, sodium stearoyl lactylate, acesulfame potassium, caramel color, sucralose.

* *Excess consumption may have a laxative effect.*

The glycemic index is a diabetic's best friend and an excellent weight loss tool. Eating foods with low GI scores help to balance blood sugar, increase energy, and promote weight loss.

Joseph's
Sugar-Free Chocolate Chip Cookies

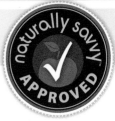

Nutrition Facts

Serving size 4 cookies (28 g)

Calories 95	Calories from fat 30
Total fat 5 g	
Saturated fat 0 g	
Trans fat 0 g	
Cholesterol 0 mg	
Sodium 40 mg	
Total carbohydrates 13 g	
Dietary fiber 1 g	
Sugars 0 g	
Protein 1 g	

INGREDIENTS: unbleached wheat flour, maltitol, canola oil, maltitol-sweetened chocolate chips (maltitol, cocoa, vanilla), natural flavors, baking soda.

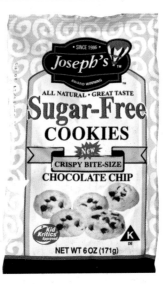

Savvy Pick
With fewer calories, fat and sodium, plus a short and sweet ingredients list, Joseph's cookies knock Murray's cookies out of the park! Murray's cookies contain risky artificial sweeteners that have been associated with serious health concerns.

Breakfast of *Champions*

Start your day with protein for a sustained feeling of fullness and better blood sugar management throughout the day. Breakfast ideas include:

- Two sunny-side-up eggs—12 g protein total, or 6 g per egg.
- Protein shake—1 scoop of protein powder provides 15 to 30 g of protein.
- Tofu—1 cup has 20 g of protein.
- Cottage cheese—½ cup has 15 g of protein.
- Nut butters –2 tablespoons have 8 g of protein.

chocolate sandwich cookies

BAD ✕ **CHOICE**

Nabisco
Oreo Cookies

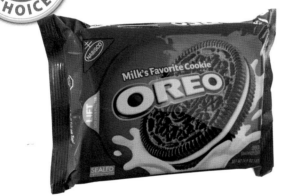

Milk's Favorite Cookie
OREO
SEALED

Nutrition Facts
Serving size 3 cookies (34 g)

Calories 160	Calories from fat 60

Total fat 7 g
Saturated fat 2 g
Trans fat 0 g
Cholesterol 0 mg
Sodium 160 mg
Total carbohydrates 25 g
Dietary fiber 1 g
Sugars 14 g
Protein 1 g

INGREDIENTS: sugar, enriched flour (wheat flour, niacin, reduced iron, thiamine mononitrate [vitamin B_1], riboflavin [vitamin B_2], folic acid), high-oleic canola oil and/or palm oil and/or canola oil and/or soybean oil, cocoa (processed with alkali), high-fructose corn syrup, cornstarch, leavening (baking soda, and/or calcium phosphate), salt, soy lecithin (emulsifier), vanillin (an artificial flavor), chocolate.

No more trans fat
Oreos are now free of partially hydrogenated oil (trans fat). Now if they would remove the high-fructose corn syrup, we could enjoy dipping them in a tall, cold glass of milk again, just like we did when we were kids.

Vanillin
Although listed as an "artificial flavor," vanillin is generally considered safe, as there have been few reported side effects as a result of its use. Still, most of the vanillin manufactured today is made from benzene, a known carcinogen and petroleum by-product (the same petroleum that is used to make gasoline). We still recommend avoiding it whenever possible.

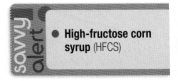

savvy alert
• **High-fructose corn syrup** (HFCS)

savvy serving Each gram of carbohydrate provides 4 calories. In a product with 130 calories per serving and 19 grams of carbohydrates, 76 of the 130 calories (that's more than half) are from carbohydrates (sugar).

Country Choice Organic
Sandwich Cremes Chocolate Cookies

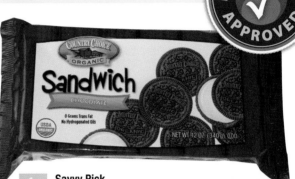

Nutrition Facts
Serving size 2 cookies (27 g)

Calories 130	Calories from fat 50
Total fat 5 g	
Saturated fat 0.5 g	
Trans fat 0 g	
Cholesterol 0 mg	
Sodium 90 mg	
Total carbohydrates 19 g	
Dietary fiber 1 g	
Sugars 11 g	
Protein 1 g	

INGREDIENTS: organic wheat flour, organic powdered sugar with organic cornstarch, organic high-oleic sunflower oil, organic sugar, organic cocoa processed with alkali, organic cane syrup, organic chocolate liquor, baking soda, organic vanilla extract, natural flavors, sea salt, soy lecithin.

Savvy Pick
The Oreo may be called "milk's favorite cookie," but we wonder if milk knows about the high-fructose corn syrup? Country Choice Organic Sandwich Cremes Chocolate Cookies are made with organic ingredients and are our top choice.

Honorable Mentions

- Newman-O's
  Crème-Filled Chocolate Cookies

- Kinnikinnick's
  KinniToos Fudge Sandwich Creme Cookies (gluten free)

- Late July
  Organic Dark Chocolate Intense & Decadent Sandwich Cookies

savvy shopping tip

You're in charge of the grocery shopping. Fill your cart with foods from the periphery of the grocery store: fresh, organic fruits and vegetables, naturally made whole grain breads (the first ingredient should read "whole grain"), lean meats and fish, and organic eggs and dairy. Treats should be just that: treats, not staples. And they should be made with wholesome ingredients.

fig bars

Nabisco
Fig Newtons

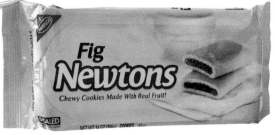

Nutrition Facts
Serving size 2 cookies (31 g)

Calories 110	Calories from fat 20
Total fat 2 g	
Saturated fat 0 g	
Trans fat 0 g	
Cholesterol 0 mg	
Sodium 130 mg	
Total carbohydrates 22 g	
Dietary fiber 1 g	
Sugars 12 g	
Protein 1 g	

Buyer beware
This product contains a lot of red flags.

📖 *Visit the glossary for an explanation of each.*

Sulfur dioxide
When buying dried fruit or products that contain dried fruit, look for the word "unsulfured" on the label. Sulfites, a group of preservatives commonly used for dried fruit, are common allergens and can cause a variety of symptoms, including headaches and skin rashes. They can also pose problems for asthmatics.

Sulfites
According to the FDA, approximately one out of every 100 people is sensitive to sulfites (also spelled sulphites). Reactions can range from mild to life threatening.

INGREDIENTS: unbleached enriched flour (wheat flour, niacin, reduced iron, thiamine mononitrate [vitamin B_1], riboflavin [vitamin B_2], folic acid), figs, high-fructose corn syrup, corn syrup, sugar, soybean oil, whey (from milk), partially hydrogenated cottonseed oil, salt, baking soda, cultured dextrose, calcium lactate, malic acid, soy lecithin, natural and artificial flavor, sulfur dioxide added to preserve freshness.

savvy alert

- **High-fructose corn syrup** (HFCS)
- **Partially hydrogenated oil** *trans fat*
- **Artificial flavor**
- **Sulfur dioxide** *sulfites*

fiber flop

Fiber-rich food (providing at least 4 grams per serving) promotes satiety and slows the absorption of carbohydrates from food. Nabisco's Fig Newton has only 1 gram of fiber, whereas a large fresh fig contains 2 grams of fiber and other important nutrients.

Barbara's
Fig Bars—Whole Wheat

naturally savvy
APPROVED

Nutrition Facts
Serving size 1 bar (38 g)

Calories 110	Calories from fat 5
Total fat 0.5 g	
Saturated fat 0 g	
Trans fat 0 g	
Cholesterol 0 mg	
Sodium 50 mg	
Total carbohydrates 25 g	
Dietary fiber 2 g	
Sugars 15 g	
Protein 1 g	

INGREDIENTS: fig filling (fig paste, pineapple juice concentrate, citric acid), pineapple juice syrup, whole wheat flour, whole barley flour, date paste, fig paste, raisin juice concentrate, expeller-pressed canola oil, baking soda, soy lecithin, salt.

Savvy Pick
It's nice to see that Barbara's Fig Bars list "figs" as the first ingredient, so you get a whole lotta fig with each bite. Plus, they're made with whole grain flours. Seven grams larger than Nabisco's Fig Newtons, they have the same number of calories but half the sodium. The fact that they're wheat and gluten free means that even more people are able to enjoy them.

Honorable Mention
❖ Newman's Own Organics
   Fig Newmans

D-I-Y Cookies

Boost the nutritional value of your home baked cookies by adding:

Ground flax—an easy way to increase the fiber and omega-3 fatty acids in your snack.
Cinnamon—a blood sugar stabilizer that just happens to taste delicious.
Nut butter—boosts the protein and adds some minerals.

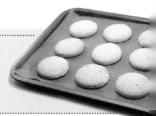

ginger snaps

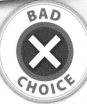
BAD ✗ CHOICE

Nabisco
Ginger Snaps

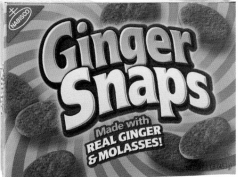

Nutrition Facts
Serving size 4 cookies (28 g)

Calories 120	Calories from fat 20

Total fat 2.5 g	
Saturated fat 0 g	
Trans fat 0 g	
Cholesterol 0 mg	
Sodium 190 mg	
Total carbohydrates 23 g	
Dietary fiber 0 g	
Sugars 11 g	
Protein 1 g	

INGREDIENTS: enriched flour (wheat flour, niacin, reduced iron, thiamine mononitrate [vitamin B$_1$], riboflavin [vitamin B$_2$], folic acid), sugar, molasses preserved with sulfur dioxide, partially hydrogenated soybean oil, leavening (baking soda, calcium phosphate), ginger, salt, soy lecithin (emulsifier).

Ginger
Zingiber officinale, commonly known as ginger, is an herb that has been used as a food additive for more than 4,000 years and for medicinal purposes for more than 2,000 years. Famous for its impact on nausea, morning sickness, and motion sickness, ginger has also been known to relieve symptoms of the common cold.

Partially hydrogenated oil *trans fat*
The FDA estimates that just reducing the amount of trans fats in foods would prevent 4,200 heart attack deaths annually.

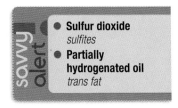

savvy alert
- **Sulfur dioxide**
  sulfites
- **Partially hydrogenated oil**
  trans fat

Pamela's Simplebites
Ginger Mini Snapz

Nutrition Facts
Serving size 4 cookies (25 g)

Calories 115	Calories from fat 35
Total fat 4 g	
Saturated fat 2 g	
Trans fat 0 g	
Cholesterol 5 mg	
Sodium 170 mg	
Total carbohydrates 20 g	
Dietary fiber 0.5 g	
Sugars 12 g	
Protein 1 g	

INGREDIENTS: rice flour base (brown rice flour, white rice flour, tapioca starch, sweet rice flour, xanthan gum), molasses, brown sugar, organic natural evaporated cane sugar, non-hydrogenated palm oil, eggs, ginger spice, gluten-free vanilla flavor, cinnamon, baking soda, sea salt, cloves.

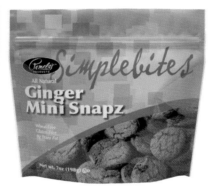

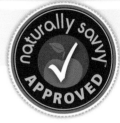

Savvy Pick
This recipe was created by Pamela herself (yes, she does exist!). To ensure her ginger snaps would sing with flavor, she created a delectable mini cookie with the perfect blend of flavor + crunch, all without trans fats or preservatives.

Honorable Mentions
✤ Mary's Gone Crackers
  Love Cookies—Ginger Snaps (wheat free, gluten free)

✤ Glow
  Gingersnap Cookies

Gluten-free Grains

Gluten-free grains do not contain gliadin, the form of protein found in gluten that is problematic for those with gluten sensitivity and celiac disease. Flour for baking can be produced from gluten-free grains, nuts, and seeds. Check bulk food and natural products stores for amaranth flour, arrowroot flour, rice flour, buckwheat flour, organic cornmeal, quinoa flour, almond flour, and tapioca flour. Store flours in the refrigerator or freezer to keep them fresh.

peanut butter sandwich cookies

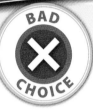

Nabisco
Nutter Butter

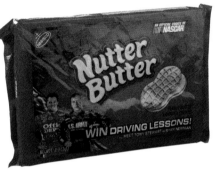

Partially hydrogenated oil
trans fat

These unhealthy fats raise triglyceride levels. Triglycerides are a type of fat found in your blood, and a high triglyceride level may contribute to hardening of the arteries (atherosclerosis) or thickening of the artery walls, which increases the risk of stroke, diabetes, heart attack, and heart disease.

Hydrogenated oils

This product contains both hydrogenated and partially hydrogenated oils (trans fats). When hydrogenated oil appears on its own in the ingredients list, the only guarantee that the product is trans-fat free is if it's listed as "fully hydrogenated."

Soybean oil

After palm oil, soybean oil is the second most widely used oil worldwide, accounting for 23 percent of the total production of oils and fats. It's popular because it's cheap, has a high smoke point, and has little flavor—an advantage because it won't interfere with the taste of the food. In supermarkets, it's often sold as "vegetable oil."

Nutrition Facts
Serving size 2 cookies (28 g)

Calories 130	Calories from fat 45
Total fat 5 g	
Saturated fat 1.5 g	
Trans fat 0 g	
Cholesterol 0 mg	
Sodium 110 mg	
Total carbohydrates 20 g	
Dietary fiber Less than 1 g	
Sugars 8 g	
Protein 2 g	

INGREDIENTS: unbleached enriched flour (wheat flour, niacin, reduced iron, thiamine mononitrate, riboflavin, folic acid), sugar, peanut butter (peanuts, corn syrup solids, hydrogenated rapeseed and/or cottonseed and/or soybean oils, peanut oil, salt), soybean oil and/or palm oil, graham flour (whole grain wheat flour), high-fructose corn syrup, partially hydrogenated cottonseed oil, salt, leavening (baking soda and/or calcium phosphate), cornstarch, soy lecithin (emulsifier), vanillin (artificial flavor).

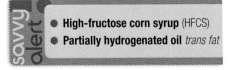

- **High-fructose corn syrup** (HFCS)
- **Partially hydrogenated oil** *trans fat*

savvy tip If you or someone you know has a peanut allergy, a great-tasting peanut butter alternative is SunButter. Completely free of peanuts and tree nuts, it's derived from sunflower seeds but looks and tastes like peanut butter. *Visit www.sunbutter.com for more information.*

Back to Nature
Peanut Butter Creme Cookies

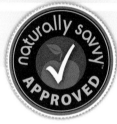

Nutrition Facts
Serving size 2 cookies (26 g)

Calories 130	Calories from fat 45
Total fat 5 g	
Saturated fat 1 g	
Trans fat 0 g	
Cholesterol 0 mg	
Sodium 95 mg	
Total carbohydrates 18 g	
Dietary fiber 1 g	
Sugars 8 g	
Protein 2 g	

INGREDIENTS: unbleached wheat flour, evaporated cane juice, peanut butter (peanuts, salt), whole grain rolled oats, safflower oil, palm oil, partially defatted peanut flour, brown rice syrup, sea salt, leavening (baking soda, monocalcium phosphate), soy lecithin, natural flavor.

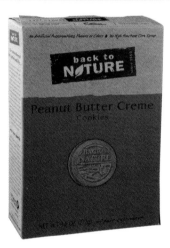

Savvy Pick
Unlike Nabisco Nutter Butter, Back to Nature is free of trans fat and high-fructose corn syrup. Also, Back to Nature's peanut butter is made from just peanuts and salt. Clearly it's the savvy option.

Peanut Allergies

The incidence of peanut allergies in North American children has doubled in the past decade, and while it isn't known why they're becoming more common, theories include overexposure to peanut proteins from skin creams containing peanut oil and exposure to foods that have a similar protein, such as soy. Ironically, peanut allergies are much less common in other parts of the world, including Asia, where peanuts are a major food source.

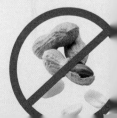

animal cookies

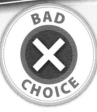

BAD X CHOICE

Nabisco Snak-Saks
Barnum's Animals Crackers

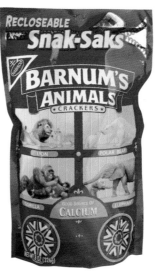

Partially hydrogenated oil
trans fat
A 2011 study concluded that most of the trans fats in our food are found in baked goods, such as cookies. Forty percent of the sixty products examined contained trans fats higher than 2 percent.

Partially hydrogenated oils
trans fats
Food companies are exploring various options for replacing trans fats in foods. Since almost any other type of fat is better than trans fat, this is mostly a step in the right direction.

History lesson
Animal crackers have been a part of U.S. cookie history for a long time: they were first imported from England in the late 1800s.

Nutrition Facts
Serving size Approx. 18 crackers (31 g)

Calories 140	Calories from fat 35
Total fat 4 g	
Saturated fat 1 g	
Trans fat 0 g	
Cholesterol 0 mg	
Sodium 150 mg	
Total carbohydrates 24 g	
Dietary fiber 1 g	
Sugars 8 g	
Protein 2 g	

INGREDIENTS: enriched flour (wheat flour, niacin, reduced iron, thiamine mononitrate, riboflavin, folic acid), high-fructose corn syrup, sugar, soybean oil, yellow corn flour, partially hydrogenated cottonseed oil, calcium carbonate (source of calcium), baking soda, salt, soy lecithin (emulsifier), natural and artificial flavors.

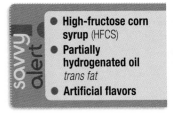

savvy alert

- **High-fructose corn syrup** (HFCS)
- **Partially hydrogenated oil** *trans fat*
- **Artificial flavors**

savvy tip

Portion control can be learned from a young age. Encourage kids to count out the serving sizes listed on the Nutrition Facts panel. In this case, Barbara's Snackimals serving size is a generous ten cookies. They'll learn to control their appetite and improve their counting skills at the same time.

Barbara's Snackimals
Animal Cookies—Vanilla

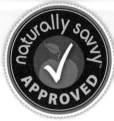

Nutrition Facts
Serving size 10 cookies (30 g)

Calories 110	Calories from fat 35

Total fat 4 g

    Saturated fat 0 g

    Trans fat 0 g

Cholesterol 0 mg

Sodium 65 mg

Total carbohydrates 17 g

    Dietary fiber 0 g

    Sugars 5 g

Protein 2 g

INGREDIENTS: organic unbleached wheat flour, unsulphured molasses, organic expeller pressed sunflower or safflower oil, natural vanilla with other natural flavors, sea salt, soy lecithin, baking soda, aluminum free baking powder (non-GMO corn starch, baking soda, monocalcium phosphate).

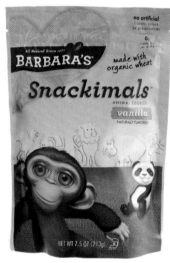

Savvy Pick
This is no time to monkey around—there shouldn't be any HFCS, trans fats, or artificial flavors in cookies made for children. You are better off with Barbara's Snackimals.

Honorable Mentions
❖ Jo-sef
   Animal Cookies
❖ KinniKritters
   Animal Cookies (gluten free)

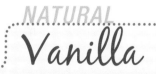

NATURAL
Vanilla

Real vanilla is the world's most labor-intensive agricultural crop. It can take three years before vanilla vines flower, and then the vanilla beans have to cure and dry to develop their distinct flavor. Added to that, vanilla is in high demand for foods and fragrances, so it's no surprise that cheaper synthetics are used more often. In fact, a whopping 98 percent of the vanilla used for flavor and fragrance is synthetic.

oatmeal raisin cookies

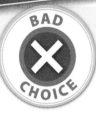

BAD **CHOICE**

Keebler Country Style
Oatmeal Cookies Baked with Raisins

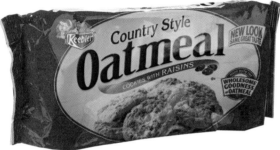

Country Style
Oatmeal
COOKIES WITH RAISINS
NEW LOOK SAME GREAT TASTE
WHOLESOME GOODNESS = OATMEAL

Nutrition Facts
Serving size 2 cookies (28 g)

Calories 130	Calories from fat 50
Total fat 6 g	
Saturated fat 2 g	
Trans fat 0 g	
Cholesterol 0 mg	
Sodium 100 mg	
Total carbohydrates 19 g	
Dietary fiber 1 g	
Sugars 8 g	
Protein 2 g	

INGREDIENTS: enriched flour (wheat flour, niacin, reduced iron, thiamine mononitrate, riboflavin, folic acid), sugar, oats, vegetable oil (soybean, palm, and palm kernel oil with TBHQ for freshness), raisins, high-fructose corn syrup. Contains 2 percent or less of: molasses, salt, baking soda, cinnamon, natural flavor, egg, whey protein concentrate, soy lecithin.

TBHQ
This preservative is sprayed directly onto foods or its packaging to avoid changes to flavor and color.

Is oatmeal gluten free?
Oatmeal is gluten free, but because it's often grown in the same fields as wheat (which contains gluten), it can become contaminated with gluten. Products containing oatmeal that are guaranteed to be gluten free will include that information on the label. Both Glutenfreeda and Bakery on Main sell certified gluten-free instant oatmeal.

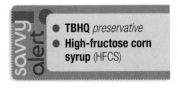

savvy alert
- **TBHQ** *preservative*
- **High-fructose corn syrup** (HFCS)

Matt's
Real Oatmeal Raisin Cookies

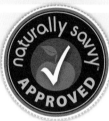

Nutrition Facts
Serving size 1 cookie (30 g)

Calories 130	Calories from fat 60

Total fat 7 g	
Saturated fat 1.5 g	
Trans fat 0 g	
Cholesterol 5 mg	
Sodium 70 mg	
Total carbohydrates 17 g	
Dietary fiber 2 g	
Sugars 9 g	
Protein 1.7 g	

INGREDIENTS: oatmeal, raisins, baking oil (palm, soybean, canola), unbleached wheat flour, brown sugar, sugar, fresh eggs, molasses, malt, cinnamon, vanilla, baking soda, salt, nutmeg, allspice.

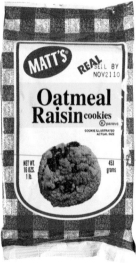

Savvy Pick

Matt's is one smart cookie. A Matt's cookie is equivalent to two Keebler cookies, but don't let the serving size fool you. In addition, sugar is listed as the fifth ingredient, rather than within the top three, and there's no high-fructose corn syrup. For all of these reasons, Matt receives our Savvy Seal of Approval™.

Honorable Mention

❖ Mary's Gone Crackers
   *"N'Oatmeal" Raisin Love Cookies
   (gluten free)*

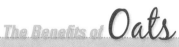

The Benefits of Oats

Oats have many health benefits. They are a whole grain low in fat and rich in dietary fiber, B vitamins, and minerals. The soluble fibers they contain bind to LDL cholesterol (the "bad" kind), helping to reduce the risk of cardiovascular disease, and they keep you feeling full longer than refined grains. Oats also help stabilize blood sugar. If you have high cholesterol or want to shed a few pounds, include oatmeal on your breakfast menu regularly.

chocolate

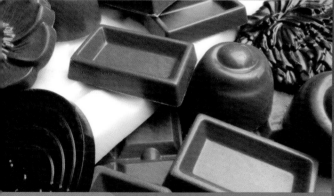

- ✤ Caramel nut chocolate bar
- ✤ Coated chocolate candy
- ✤ Chocolate peanut butter cups
- ✤ Coconut almond bar
- ✤ Chocolate covered caramels
- ✤ Chocolate covered peanuts
- ✤ Chocolate covered crispy wafer bars

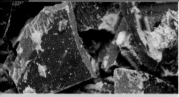

THE PROS & CONS of Chocolate

PROS

+ Chocolate is a rich source of antioxidants (polyphenols). The darker the chocolate, the better it is for you.

+ Chocolate contains theobromine, which has been shown to help prevent asthma attacks.

+ Chocolate's antioxidants can improve your memory.

+ Chocolate provides energy when you're on the go.

+ Chocolate has been shown to help prevent cardiovascular disease, stroke, and type 2 diabetes.

+ Chocolate can play a role in promoting longevity.

CONS

+ Chocolate can cause weight gain if eaten in excess.

+ Chocolate is addictive!

+ Remember, sometimes you can have too much of a good thing.

WORST INGREDIENTS we found in **chocolate**

+ Artificial colors
+ Artificial flavors
+ High-fructose corn syrup (HFCS)
+ Partially hydrogenated oils (trans fats)
+ Sodium metabisulfite
+ Sulfur dioxide
+ TBHQ

also **beware** of

+ Annatto color
+ Caramel color
+ Carrageenan

+ Hydrolyzed milk protein
+ PGPR (polyglycerol polyricinoleate)

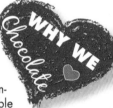

It's no wonder chocolate is considered by many to be the undisputed champion of all snack foods. After all, it combines a delectable indulgence with real health benefits, making it a not-so-guilty pleasure that is not only hard to resist but also can be downright addictive.

In the past, chocolate was generally seen as an unhealthy junk food. Nowadays, thanks to new research, many people are rediscovering the health benefits of chocolate.

WHY WE Chocolate

Reasons You Might Be Craving
. . . Chocolate

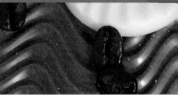

Have you ever craved chocolate? It might have something to do with the three hundred plus compounds that have been identified and isolated in chocolate.

ENERGY
Chocolate contains sugar and caffeine, both of which provide immediate "feel good" energy.

LOVE DRUG
The phenylethylamine (PEA) is a natural antidepressant that can help improve one's mood quickly. This explains why chocolate is considered an aphrodisiac.

MAGNESIUM
Sometimes cravings for chocolate are due to a deficiency in the mineral magnesium. Magnesium is also found in nuts, pumpkin seeds, spinach, bran, beans, and brown rice. Depleted during menstruation, low magnesium may also be the reason for monthly chocolate cravings among premenstrual women. Some believe that women crave chocolate as the body's way of stocking up on magnesium before menstruation.

STRESS
Chocolate also contains the amino acid tryptophan, an important factor in the production of the mood-modulating neurotransmitter serotonin, which diminishes anxiety, helping you to relax.

PAIN RELIEF
Chocolate triggers the release of endorphins, natural pain relievers that provide an all-over feel-good state.

health alert!

Caffeine is a natural compound found in coffee, tea, AND **cocoa beans.**

- 1 ounce of dark chocolate contains about 20 milligrams of caffeine.
- 1 ounce of milk chocolate contains about 6 milligrams of caffeine, or about the same amount as a cup of decaf coffee.
- 1 ounce of white chocolate contains less than 2 milligrams of caffeine.

In comparison, an average chocolate bar contains about 30 milligrams of caffeine and the average cup of coffee approximately 80 to 155 milligrams. To get the caffeine equivalent of one cup of coffee, you would have to eat anywhere from two to five chocolate bars.

Chocolate Trivia

Q : Why does some chocolate turn white?

A : When milk chocolate produces white spots on its surface, it is said to have bloomed. Blooming occurs when chocolate has been improperly stored or has been exposed to warm temperatures for a long time. Fortunately, it poses no health hazards—and is still good to eat!

CHOCOLATE Grows on Trees

Chocolate is made from the seeds of the tropical Theobroma cacao tree. Cocoa beans are actually the seeds of the cocoa pod, or fruit.

Once the cocoa pods are harvested, the cocoa beans are removed, fermented, and dried. They are then roasted, ground, and transformed into cocoa mass and cocoa butter—the essential ingredients for making chocolate.

Tasty Terms

COCOA MASS
The main ingredient in chocolate, cocoa mass is the product of grinding roasted cocoa nibs into a thick, dark brown paste. It is also known as cocoa solid and cocoa liquor.

COCOA BUTTER
The natural fat extracted from the cocoa bean.

COCOA POWDER
The result of drying cocoa liquor paste and grinding it to the consistency of a powder.

Why is **chocolate** healthy?

Dark chocolate is one of the richest sources of a group of antioxidants called polyphenols. A 40-gram portion of dark chocolate contains 400 to 800 milligrams of polyphenols, compared to red wine's 170 milligrams (per 100 milliliters) and an apple's 200 milligrams.

To benefit from the antioxidants in chocolate eat about 6.7 grams of dark chocolate a day—that's less than a half bar a week. Choose dairy-free chocolate with a cocoa content of 70 percent or higher.

TYPES OF **CHOCOLATE**

Whether you're hankering for dark, milk, or white chocolate, chances are there's chocolate out there with your name on it.

Dark chocolate contains cocoa butter and cocoa solids. Different varieties of dark chocolate are categorized based on the percentage of cocoa solids and the amount of sugar they contain. The healthiest dark chocolate has 70% or more cocoa.

- Unsweetened chocolate, also known as bitter chocolate or baking chocolate, contains no sugar and 41 percent to 50 percent cocoa liquor. It's bitter, so it's primarily used for cooking.
- Bittersweet chocolate contains little sugar and at least 35 percent cocoa liquor.
- Semisweet chocolate contains slightly more sugar than bittersweet chocolate and has at least 35 percent cocoa liquor.
- Sweet chocolate contains the most sugar and the least amount of cocoa solids—at least 15 percent cocoa liquor.

Milk chocolate contains milk (at least 12 percent) in addition to cocoa butter, cocoa solids, sugar, and flavorings.

White chocolate contains at least 20 percent cocoa butter, sugar, milk, and vanilla but no cocoa solids.

Vegan chocolate is made with non-dairy alternatives. It's also a great option for someone who is intolerant or allergic to dairy products.

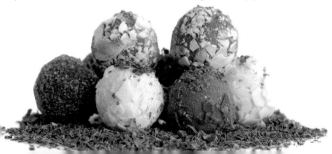

ETHICAL CHOCOLATE: **Fair Trade**

Purchasing chocolate that is labeled Fair Trade, Rainforest Alliance Certified, or UTZ certified ensures that:

- Farmers and farm workers are paid fairly.
- Farming methods protect natural resources and the environment.
- The rights and welfare of workers and the local communities are protected.

DON'T Be Misled

Good quality chocolate does not contain any of the following:

- Genetically modified ingredients (GMOs)
- Corn syrup solids
- Vegetable oils
- Chemicals such as dipotassium phosphate, sodium silicoaluminate, and PGPR
- Artificial flavor

caramel nut chocolate bar

Snickers Bar

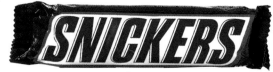

Nutrition Facts

Serving size 1 bar (2.07 oz/58.7 g)

Calories 280	Calories from fat 130
Total fat 14 g	
Saturated fat 5 g	
Trans fat 0 g	
Cholesterol 5 mg	
Sodium 140 mg	
Total carbohydrates 35 g	
Dietary fiber 1 g	
Sugars 30 g	
Protein 4 g	

INGREDIENTS: milk chocolate (sugar, cocoa butter, chocolate, skim milk, lactose, milkfat, soy lecithin, artificial flavor), peanuts, corn syrup, sugar, milkfat, skim milk, partially hydrogenated soybean oil, lactose, salt, egg whites, chocolate, artificial flavor.

Partially hydrogenated oil *trans fat*

We were very disappointed to find dangerous trans fat in a Snickers bar. The effects of trans fats are cumulative, which means that being exposed to it early on in life increases the likelihood that you can develop a chronic illness, such as heart disease, later on. Think twice before giving your child a seemingly harmless treat, such as a Snickers bar.

Artificial flavors

According to the FDA, if a company uses only a small amount of an artificial flavoring in its products, it doesn't have to specify what that ingredient is. In this case, we suspect it's vanillin.

Did you know?

Created by Mars Inc. in 1930, the Snickers bar was named after one of the beloved horses owned by the Mars family. The bar had global annual sales of more than $2 billion in 2006, becoming the most popular candy bar in the world.

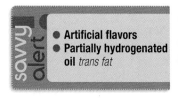

savvy alert
- **Artificial flavors**
- **Partially hydrogenated oil** *trans fat*

savvy serving To burn off a caramel nut chocolate candy bar, you must do one of the following:
• 25 minutes of jogging • 35 minutes of spinning, or • 27 minutes of stair climbing.

Jokerz Bar

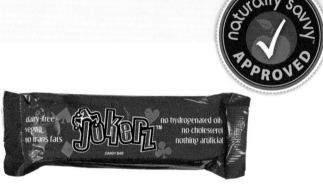

Nutrition Facts

Serving size 1 bar (2.1 oz/60 g)

Calories 280	Calories from fat 130
Total fat 15 g	
Saturated fat 6 g	
Trans fat 0 g	
Cholesterol 0 mg	
Sodium 95 mg	
Total carbohydrates 33 g	
Dietary fiber 2 g	
Sugars 22 g	
Protein 5 g	

INGREDIENTS (VEGAN): corn syrup, peanuts (dry roasted), beet sugar, evaporated cane juice, palm kernel oil, cocoa powder (natural), palm oil, rice powder (rice syrup powder, rice starch, rice flour, carrageenan), soy protein concentrate, dextrose, natural flavors, malt powder (extract of barley malt and corn), soybean lecithin, salt, carrageenan, enzyme modified soy protein.

Savvy Pick

Unfortunately, trans fat hasn't stopped Snickers from becoming one of the most loved candy bars in the world. Jokerz, however, is a yummy competitor that is free of trans fats. We felt it was the closest in taste to Snickers of the bars we tried, and although it has carrageenan, it's still the better choice. It's also vegan. For this, it gets our Savvy Seal of Approval™.

What is ...

Carrageenan

Carrageenan is an extract from seaweed that acts as a stabilizer and thickening agent in many products, including chocolate, ice cream, soups, infant formulas, and diet soda. Although it is used for many natural products, its safety for human consumption is still under investigation.

coated chocolate candy

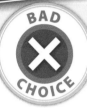

M&M's
Chocolate Candies—Milk Chocolate

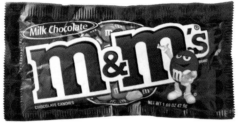

Artificial colors

Our main issue with M&M's is the array of artificial colors they contain. Even though the FDA approves them, Mars, Inc., the makers of M&M's should update their ingredients by replacing these potentially dangerous chemicals with the natural colorants that the FDA also approves.

Artificial colors

These dyes contain various chemicals and are commonly derived from petroleum—a toxic liquid oil that is also used to manufacture gasoline, asphalt, and pharmaceuticals.

Artificial flavors

The tongue can detect the differences between sweet, salty, sour, bitter, and astringent tastes. Our other senses come into play—smell, texture, and eye appeal—to determine our impression of the way a food tastes and how much we like it.

Nutrition Facts
Serving size 1 package (1.69 oz/47.9 g)

Calories 240	Calories from fat 90
Total fat 10 g	
Saturated fat 6 g	
Trans fat 0 g	
Cholesterol 5 mg	
Sodium 30 mg	
Total carbohydrates 34 g	
Dietary fiber 1 g	
Sugars 31 g	
Protein 2 g	

INGREDIENTS: milk chocolate (sugar, chocolate, cocoa butter, skim milk, milkfat, lactose, soy lecithin, salt, artificial flavors), sugar, cornstarch, less than 1 percent—corn syrup, dextrin, coloring (includes Blue 1 lake, Red 40 lake, Yellow 6, Yellow 5, Red 40, Blue 1, Blue 2 lake, Yellow 6 lake, Yellow 5 lake, Blue 2), gum acacia.

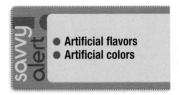

savvy alert
● Artificial flavors
● Artificial colors

savvy fact Americans eat 12 pounds of chocolate each year.

SunSpire SunDrops Original
Milk Chocolate Candies

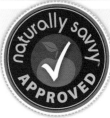

Nutrition Facts
Serving size 1 bag (1.6 oz/34 g)

Calories 180	Calories from fat 110
Total fat 12 g	
Saturated fat 7 g	
Trans fat 0 g	
Cholesterol 10 mg	
Sodium 55 mg	
Total carbohydrates 18 g	
Dietary fiber 1 g	
Sugars 16 g	
Protein 2 g	

INGREDIENTS: CENTER: dried cane juice and unsulfured molasses, whole milk powder, cocoa butter, unsweetened chocolate, non-GMO soy lecithin (emulsifier), pure natural vanilla; SHELL: dried cane juice, whole rice solids, beta-carotene color, beet juice color, and caramel color, vegetable and beeswax, pure food glaze (without sugar).

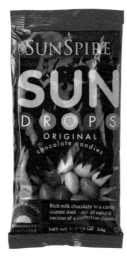

 Savvy Pick
SunSpire SunDrops taste remarkably similar to M&M's. Just looking at M&M's long list of ten artificial colors (yes, you read it right; ten different food colorants in one product) is enough to convince us that SunDrops is absolutely the better choice.

Color Your World

The colors found in natural foods indicate the nutrients they provide:

- Yellow and orange foods (like sweet potatoes and carrots) contain carotenoids that can reduce cancer risk.
- Green foods (broccoli, spinach) contain lutein, which is good for vision.
- Blue and purple foods (think berries) contain anthocyanins, which may help prevent tumor growth.
- Red foods (like tomatoes) contain lycopene, which protects against heart disease and prostate cancer.
- White foods (garlic and onions) contain flavonoids, which can help fight cancer.

chocolate peanut butter cups

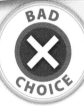

Reese's
Milk Chocolate Peanut Butter Cups

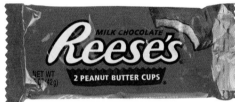

Nutrition Facts	
Serving size 1 package (1.5 oz/42 g)	

Calories 210	Calories from fat 110
Total fat 13 g	
Saturated fat 4.5 g	
Trans fat 0 g	
Cholesterol 5 mg	
Sodium 150 mg	
Total carbohydrates 24 g	
Dietary fiber 1 g	
Sugars 21 g	
Protein 5 g	

INGREDIENTS: milk chocolate (sugar, cocoa butter, chocolate, nonfat milk, milk fat, lactose, soy lecithin, PGPR, emulsifier), peanuts, sugar, dextrose, salt, TBHQ (preservative).

PGPR
The emulsifier, polyglycerol polyricinoleate is a cheap replacement for cocoa butter in chocolate bars. PGPR is made from castor oil and is often paired with the soy-based emulsifier lecithin. Although no adverse health effects have been reported for PGPR, the main reason it's used is to save companies money.

PGPR
Lowers the viscosity of chocolate, providing that creamy melt-in-your-mouth texture.

Soy lecithin
If you have an allergy to soy, watch out for soy lecithin, hydrolyzed vegetable protein, and textured vegetable protein—just a few of the many ingredients that include soy.

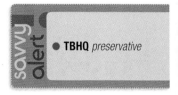

savvy alert
● **TBHQ** *preservative*

chocolate or sex? Some 50 percent of women claim to prefer chocolate to sex, according to a British survey by Cadbury.

Sun Cups
Sunflower Butter—Milk Chocolate

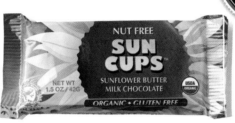

Nutrition Facts
Serving size 2 pieces (1.5 oz/42 g)

Calories 240	Calories from fat 140
Total fat 16 g	
Saturated fat 6 g	
Trans fat 0 g	
Cholesterol 5 mg	
Sodium 25 mg	
Total carbohydrates 16 g	
Dietary fiber 1 g	
Sugars 15 g	
Protein 4 g	

INGREDIENTS: milk chocolate (cane sugar, cocoa butter, whole milk powder, cocoa liquor), sunflower seed, glucose, white chocolate (cane sugar, milk powder, cocoa butter, organic soy lecithin, vanilla), cocoa butter, glucose, sea salt.

Savvy Pick
Although Sun Cups are not made with peanut butter—they are made with sunflower seeds—they are just as amazing. Made with organic nut-free sunflower butter, Sun Cups are a lifesaver for those with peanut allergies.

Honorable Mentions

❖ SunSpire
   Dark Chocolate Almond Butter Cups

❖ Newman's Own Organics
   Peanut Butter Cups

What is ... Cocoa Butter

The fat that occurs naturally in cocoa beans gives chocolate its distinctive smoothness and melt-in-the-mouth texture. Research has shown that cocoa butter, despite its high saturated fat content, does not raise blood cholesterol levels as do other saturated fats. This is due to its high stearic acid content. Stearic acid is converted in the liver to oleic acid, a heart-healthy monounsaturated fat.

coconut almond bar

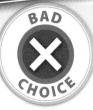

Almond Joy
Coconut & Almonds—Milk Chocolate

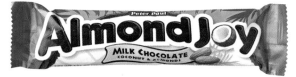

Nutrition Facts
Serving size 1 package (45 g)

Calories 220	Calories from fat 120
Total fat 13 g	
Saturated fat 8 g	
Trans fat 0 g	
Cholesterol 0 mg	
Sodium 70 mg	
Total carbohydrates 26 g	
Dietary fiber 2 g	
Sugars 20 g	
Protein 2 g	

Sodium metabisulfite and sulfur dioxide
Those with sensitivities to sulfites beware, Almond Joy contains two forms of sulfites.

Hydrolyzed milk protein (HMP)
Hydrolyzed milk protein contains glutamate, an ingredient in MSG. If you have a reaction to an Almond Joy bar, it could be due to this ingredient.

Caramel color
Food manufacturers can choose from four types of caramel coloring. Two types are safe, but the other two (Caramel III and Caramel IV) are produced with ammonia, resulting in the production of cancer-causing chemicals. Unfortunately, the type of caramel used in a product is not specified on food labels. This is the case for both conventional and natural products.

INGREDIENTS: corn syrup, milk chocolate (sugar, cocoa butter, milk, corn syrup solid, milk fat, non-fat milk, soy lecithin), coconut, sugar, almonds (roasted in cocoa butter and/or sunflower oil), 2 percent or less of partially hydrogenated vegetable oil (soybean and palm), whey, cocoa, salt, natural and artificial flavors, chocolate, soy lecithin, hydrolyzed milk protein, sodium metabisulfite, sulfur dioxide, caramel color.

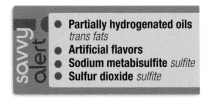

savvy alert
- **Partially hydrogenated oils** *trans fats*
- **Artificial flavors**
- **Sodium metabisulfite** *sulfite*
- **Sulfur dioxide** *sulfite*

healthy fats

The fats in coconut—called medium-chain triglycerides—are among the healthiest. Other foods containing healthy fats include salmon (wild is best), avocado, and almonds.

SunSpire
Coconut Almond Bar—Milk Chocolate

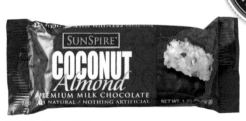

Nutrition Facts
Serving size 1 bar (1.75 oz/50 g)

Calories 260	Calories from fat 150
Total fat 16 g	
Saturated fat 12 g	
Trans fat 0 g	
Cholesterol 5 mg	
Sodium 40 mg	
Total carbohydrates 25 g	
Dietary fiber 3 g	
Sugars 13 g	
Protein 3 g	

INGREDIENTS: milk chocolate (evaporated cane juice, unsulfured molasses, whole milk powder, cocoa butter, unsweetened chocolate, non-GMO soy lecithin [emulsifier], pure natural vanilla), white rice syrup, dried unsweetened coconut, dry roasted almonds.

Savvy Pick
SunSpire's bar is larger, so it's higher in fat and calories than Almond Joy but lower in sodium and sugar. Trans-fat free and sulfite free, SunSpire also uses non-GMO soy lecithin as an emulsifier. For all of this, we are overjoyed.

Refer to chapter 2 for an explanation of GMOs.

Honorable Mention
+ Crispy Cat
   Toasted Almond Bar

Nuts for Coconuts

Coconuts are a special fruit rich in fiber and nutrients; but it's the oil that is attributed with many of its healing properties. Though mostly saturated, coconut oil's medium-chain triglycerides (MCTs) are very different from the long-chain fatty acids found in most other foods. MCTs reduce the risk of heart disease and promote a healthy weight, whereas most other fats contribute to weight gain. For baking and frying, use unrefined, organic coconut oil. *For recipes using coconut, visit www.naturallysavvy.com/recipes.*

chocolate covered caramels

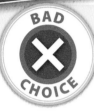

Rolo
Chewy Caramels in Milk Chocolate

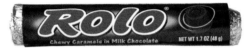

Chewy Caramels in Milk Chocolate   NET WT 1.7 OZ (48 g)

Rolo "no-no"
This is one of the worst products in our chocolate chapter. It contains both trans fats and high-fructose corn syrup.

High-fructose corn syrup
In 2006, the U.S. government gave the corn industry $4,920,813,719 in subsidies, allowing them to sell their crops very cheaply and still make profits. It's no wonder food manufacturers prefer to use this sweetener over real sugar.

Artificial flavor (vanillin)
You may notice that artificial flavors are listed twice in the ingredients (which we usually flag in red), but in this case, they're referring to vanillin (a yellow flag). While vanillin is an ingredient in the vanilla bean, most of the vanillin used in processed food is synthetic. Artificial vanilla, often denoted as "vanillin, artificial flavor," is mostly produced from guaicol, a petrochemical. Nevertheless, we have not come across any specific ill effects other than migraine headaches from its consumption.

Nutrition Facts
Serving size 1 package (1.7 oz/48 g)

Calories 220	Calories from fat 90

Total fat 10 g	
Saturated fat 7 g	
Trans fat 0 g	
Cholesterol 5 mg	
Sodium 80 mg	
Total carbohydrates 33 g	
Dietary fiber 0 g	
Sugars 29 g	
Protein 2 g	

INGREDIENTS: milk chocolate (sugar, non-fat milk, cocoa butter, chocolate, lactose (milk), milk fat, soy lecithin, PGPR [emulsifier], vanillin, artificial flavor), sugar, corn syrup, high-fructose corn syrup, partially hydrogenated vegetable oil (palm kernel and soybean oil), milk, salt, sodium bicarbonate, and vanillin, artificial flavor.

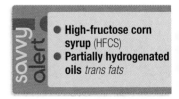

savvy alert

- **High-fructose corn syrup** (HFCS)
- **Partially hydrogenated oils** *trans fats*

savvy serving

Your fat intake should constitute about 25 percent of your calories. That means if you eat about 2,000 calories a day, no more than 500 calories should come from fats.

Newman's Own Organics
Milk Chocolate Caramel Cups

Nutrition Facts
Serving size 1 package (1.2 oz/34 g)

Calories 160	Calories from fat 70
Total fat 8 g	
Saturated fat 5 g	
Trans fat 0 g	
Cholesterol 5 mg	
Sodium 40 mg	
Total carbohydrates 21 g	
Dietary fiber 0 g	
Sugars 16 g	
Protein 2 g	

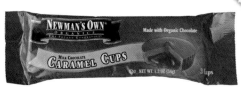

INGREDIENTS: organic milk chocolate (organic evaporated cane juice, organic cocoa butter, organic whole milk powder, organic chocolate liquor, organic soy lecithin [emulsifier], organic vanilla), organic liquid caramel (organic corn syrup, organic cane sugar, organic nonfat milk, organic heavy cream, organic butter [cream, salt], salt, sodium citrate, organic vanilla extract, organic soy lecithin [emulsifier], and vitamin E [mixed tocopherols; preservative]).

Savvy Pick
This was an easy one. Newman's Own Organics Milk Chocolate Caramel Cups are made with organic ingredients, are lower in fat and calories than Rolo, are free of high-fructose corn syrup and trans fats, and are absolutely delicious.

Honorable Mention

❖ Newman's Own Organics
Dark Chocolate Caramel Cups

Why is Chocolate Poisonous to Dogs?

Chocolate contains theobromine and caffeine, members of a class of compounds called methylxanthines. In animals, theobromine can induce cardiac arrhythmias and seizures. The toxic dose of theobromine (and caffeine) for pets is 100 to 200 milligrams per kilogram (2.2 pounds). However, the American Society for the Prevention of Cruelty to Animals (ASPCA) has reported problems at doses as low as 20 milligrams per kilogram.

chocolate covered peanuts

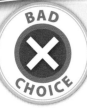

BAD ✗ **CHOICE**

Nestlé Goobers
Fresh Roasted Peanuts—Milk Chocolate

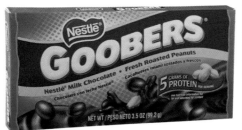

TBHQ
Antioxidants should be a good thing, but some synthetic antioxidants like TBHQ, BHA, and BHT that are used as food additives to prevent the rancidity of fats and oils can have unpleasant side effects. All three have been associated with hyperactivity in children.

Leader in preservatives
China is currently the world's leading supplier of preservatives and food flavorings. The three most common food additives that the United States imports from China are citric acid, sorbic acid, and vanillin.

Savvy fact
In October 2007, Mayu Yamamoto, a 26-year-old Japanese researcher from the International Medical Center of Japan, developed a way to extract vanillin from cow dung. She won an Ig Nobel prize for her efforts!

Nutrition Facts
Serving size 1.3 oz (1 whole bag)

Calories 210	Calories from fat 120
Total fat 14 g	
Saturated fat 5 g	
Trans fat 0 g	
Cholesterol 5 mg	
Sodium 15 mg	
Total carbohydrates 22 g	
Dietary fiber 2 g	
Sugars 18 g	
Protein 5 g	

INGREDIENTS: milk chocolate (sugar, cocoa butter, milk, chocolate, lactose, milkfat, soy lecithin, vanillin [artificial flavor]), peanuts, sugar, cocoa processed with alkali, tapioca dextrin, confectioner's glaze (lac-resin), citric acid, TBHQ.

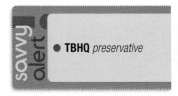

savvy alert

● **TBHQ** *preservative*

savvy serving The average chocolate bar provides 13 grams of fat. Keep this in mind when you are craving that midafternoon pick-me-up.

SunRidge Farms
Chocolate Toffee Peanuts

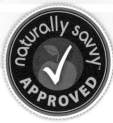

Nutrition Facts

Serving size 6 pieces (40 g/1.4 oz)

Calories 200	Calories from fat 100
Total fat 11 g	
Saturated fat 5 g	
Trans fat 0 g	
Cholesterol 5 mg	
Sodium 45 mg	
Total carbohydrates 24 g	
Dietary fiber 1 g	
Sugars 22 g	
Protein 3 g	

INGREDIENTS: milk chocolate coating (dehydrated cane juice, cocoa butter, unsweetened chocolate, whole milk powder, soy lecithin [added as an emulsifier], natural vanilla), butter toffee peanuts (evaporated cane juice, peanuts, butter [cream, {milk}, salt, annatto color {added seasonally}], salt), pure food glaze.

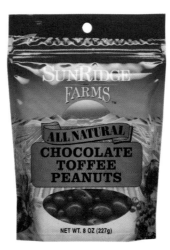

Savvy Pick
Even though SunRidge Farms Chocolate Toffee Peanuts has 30 more milligrams of sodium per serving, we chose it because it doesn't contain vanillin and TBHQ—synthetic ingredients you can do without.

Natural Peanut Butter

Many conventional brands of peanut butter contain partially hydrogenated fat (trans fat). Natural peanut butter is made with just peanuts and maybe a sprinkle of salt. You'll notice a layer of oil sitting on top of the peanut butter when you open it, so give it a good stir before spreading. Or turn the container upside down for a minute or two prior to opening it. The separation is due to the lack of added fat.

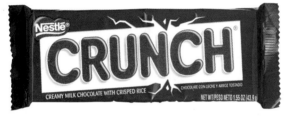

chocolate covered crispy wafer bars

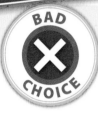

Nestlé Crunch
Milk Chocolate with Crisped Rice

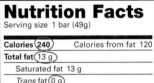

Nutrition Facts
Serving size 1 bar (49g)

Calories 240	Calories from fat 120
Total fat 13 g	
Saturated fat 13 g	
Trans fat 0 g	
Cholesterol 0 mg	
Sodium 65 mg	
Total carbohydrates 32 g	
Dietary fiber 1 g	
Sugars 21 g	
Protein 3 g	

INGREDIENTS: sugar, wheat flour, hydrogenated coconut oil, hydrogenated palm kernel oil, alkalized cocoa, nonfat milk, crisped rice (rice flour, sugar, barley malt, salt), one percent or less of each: high-fructose corn syrup, soy lecithin, artificial vanilla flavor, salt, baking soda, lactic acid esters, TBHQ and citric acid (preservatives), ground peanuts.

Hydrogenated coconut oil
This is not the same thing as unrefined, organic extra-virgin coconut oil (the type we recommend). Hydrogenated coconut oil may contain trans fats and other harmful toxins and should be strictly avoided.

Hydrogenated palm kernel oil
Hydrogenated oil is a way for food companies to extend the shelf life of oil in a product that would normally (or should we say, naturally) go rancid.

Artificial vanilla flavor
This is just another way to say "vanillin."

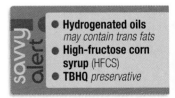

savvy alert
- **Hydrogenated oils** *may contain trans fats*
- **High-fructose corn syrup** (HFCS)
- **TBHQ** *preservative*

eat it raw

Raw chocolate is one of the healthiest foods found in nature. It's often sold as cacao nibs, which have not been processed or heated. It doesn't exactly taste like chocolate as we know it, but more like a cross between a coffee bean and chocolate.

Q.bel
Crispy Rice Milk Chocolate Wafer Bar

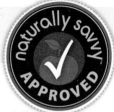

naturally savvy ✓ APPROVED

Nutrition Facts

Serving size 2 bars (32 g)

Calories 180	Calories from fat 100
Total fat 11 g	
Saturated fat 7 g	
Trans fat 0 g	
Cholesterol 5 mg	
Sodium 25 mg	
Total carbohydrates 16 g	
Dietary fiber 0 g	
Sugars 12 g	
Protein 2 g	

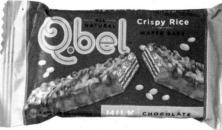

Savvy Pick

Q.bel is a smaller-size bar (let's call it portion control) and is lower in sodium than Nestlé Crunch. Throw in some abbreviations—HFCS and TBHQ—and Nestlé gets a big thumbs-down for this one.

INGREDIENTS: milk chocolate (sugar, cocoa butter, whole milk powder, chocolate liquor, soy lecithin [an emulsifier], natural vanilla), non-hydrogenated palm oil, sugar, wheat flour, crisped rice (rice flour, sugar, malt, wheat gluten, salt, canola lecithin [an emulsifier]), low-fat cocoa powder, skimmed milk powder, non-hydrogenated coconut oil, egg yolk, canola lecithin, salt, caramel color.

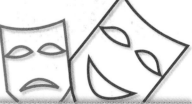

Mood Food

Chocolate is high in phenylethylamine (PEA), which is thought to help create feelings of attraction and excitement. Dark chocolate also releases both endorphins and serotonin. Each acts as a natural antidepressant and can suppress appetite.

cakes & other desserts

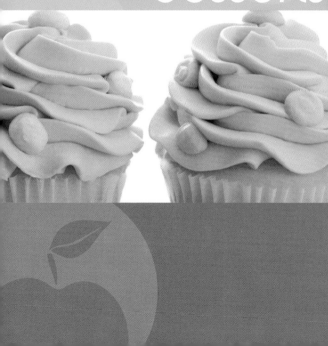

8

- ✤ Apple pie
- ✤ Pie shells
- ✤ Cheesecake
- ✤ Brownies
- ✤ Cinnamon buns—Refrigerated dough
- ✤ Cupcakes
- ✤ Donuts
- ✤ Chocolate cake mix
- ✤ Ready-to-spread frosting
- ✤ Whipped dessert toppings

How It All Began

There's a theory that the ancient Greeks are the source of one of the most common birthday traditions of all time: lighting birthday candles. Long ago, it was believed that the smoke from the burning candles had the ability to carry prayers to the gods. This tradition has evolved over time to become the much-encouraged silent birthday wish made before blowing out the candles.

NURSERY RHYME

The history of the "Pat-a-cake" nursery rhyme has been traced back as far as 1698!

**Pat-a-cake, pat-a-cake,
baker's man,
Bake me a cake
as fast as you can.
Pat it and prick it
and mark it with B,
And put it in the oven for
baby and me.**

WORST INGREDIENTS

we found in
cakes & other desserts

- Artificial colors
- Artificial flavors
- BHA and BHT
- High-fructose corn syrup
- Partially hydrogenated vegetable oil (trans fat)
- Polysorbate 60
- Polysorbate 80
- Sodium benzoate
- Sodium metabisulfite
- TBHQ

also **beware** of

- Caramel color
- Carrageenan
- Hydrogenated oil
  (may contain trans fats)
- Margarine
  (may contain trans fats)
- Potassium sorbate

- Propylene glycol
- Sodium caseinate
- Sodium stearoyl lactylate
- Sorbitan monostearate
- Titanium dioxide
- Vegetable shortening
  (may contain trans fats)

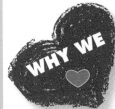

WHY WE — Cakes & other desserts

Cake is often the dessert of choice for special occasions, particularly weddings, anniversaries, and birthdays. With professional cake decorating events, reality TV shows based entirely around the art of creating cakes that look like masterpieces, and cupcake shops opening up on every corner, the cake and cupcake industry has exploded.

Reasons You Might Be Craving

. . . Cakes & Other Desserts

ADDICTIVE

For one thing, sugar is addictive. Nearly all simple sugars are metabolized quickly and disrupt insulin levels. What's more, sugar suppresses the immune system.

TO FEEL GOOD

Carbohydrate-heavy treats such as donuts and cakes raise our blood sugar levels and trigger the release of insulin, which messes with our brain chemicals. Sugar allows tryptophan to quickly enter the brain, where it is used to make the feel-good neurotransmitter serotonin. So eating carbohydrates literally makes you feel good—but it's a quick fix.

LOW ENERGY

Likewise, sugar spikes blood sugar levels, but here too the instant energy is temporary. Giving in to sugar cravings can have negative consequences down the road, such as weight gain.

Sweet "I Do's": How Far We Have Come

Early wedding cakes took on many forms and customs. One we think is particularly interesting took place in medieval England, where wedding cakes were made of spiced buns and built very tall. According to custom, if the bride and groom could easily kiss above the cake, it meant they would lead a successful life together.

Did You Know?

According to the Wedding and Bridal Association of America, the average cost of a wedding cake is $543!

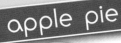

apple pie

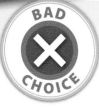

BAD CHOICE

Mrs. Smith's
Deep Dish Apple Pie

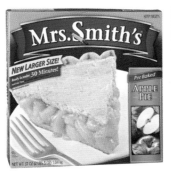

Unhealthy ingredients
What's more American than apple pie? Unfortunately, most apple pie is now often loaded with high-fructose corn syrup, trans fats, and preservatives. This product is a good example.

Margarine and shortening
These ingredients indicate that Mrs. Smith's Deep Dish Apple Pie likely contains trans fats.

Sodium benzoate
Studies suggest that sodium benzoate is to blame for hyperactivity in some children.

Why acids?
Acids are used in foods to make flavors taste sharper. They can also be used as preservatives and antioxidants. Citric acid, for example, is naturally derived from citrus fruits and can add a nice tang to a product's flavor.

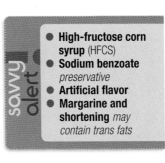

savvy alert

- **High-fructose corn syrup** (HFCS)
- **Sodium benzoate** *preservative*
- **Artificial flavor**
- **Margarine and shortening** *may contain trans fats*

Nutrition Facts
Serving size 1/10 of a pie (128 g or 4.5 oz)

Calories 290	Calories from fat 120
Total fat 13 g	
Saturated fat 6 g	
Trans fat 0 g	
Cholesterol 0 mg	
Sodium 330 mg	
Total carbohydrates 41 g	
Dietary fiber 2 g	
Sugars 18 g	
Protein 3 g	

INGREDIENTS: sliced apples, wheat flour, water, high-fructose corn syrup, margarine (palm oil, water, soybean oil, salt, vegetable mono- and diglycerides, soy lecithin, sodium benzoate [a preservative], citric acid, natural and artificial flavor, beta-carotene [color], vitamin A (palmitate added), vegetable shortening (palm oil and soybean oil with mono- and diglycerides), corn syrup, brown sugar. Contains 2 percent or less of each of the following: modified food starch, salt, dextrose, ascorbic acid, citric acid, yeast, spice, calcium chloride, baking soda, bleached wheat flour with malted barley, preserved with potassium sorbate and sodium benzoate.

savvy tip The morning after a night of indulging in a decadent dessert, drink a glass of warm water with lemon before eating or drinking. This will help stimulate digestion and elimination—in other words, it helps to clean out the pipes.

Wholly Wholesome
Truly Natural Apple Pie

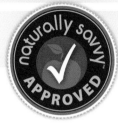

Nutrition Facts	
Serving size ⅛ of the pie (122 g or 4.3 oz)	
Calories 330	Calories from fat 140
Total fat 15 g	
Saturated fat 8 g	
Trans fat 0 g	
Cholesterol 0 mg	
Sodium 135 mg	
Total carbohydrates 45 g	
Dietary fiber 1 g	
Sugars 24 g	
Protein 2 g	

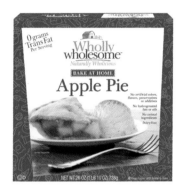

INGREDIENTS: apples, organic cane sugar, water, organic wheat flour, vegetable oil (palm oil, soybean oil), organic whole wheat flour, rice starch, sea salt, cinnamon, nutmeg, allspice.

Savvy Pick
We're pretty sure that mom's apple pie didn't have high-fructose corn syrup in it, so why is it used in Mrs. Smith's? Because it's cheap. Wholly Wholesome is made with organic flour and real, organic cane sugar. And when you're comparing apples to apples (pies, that is), nothing tastes like the real thing. Look for it in the frozen foods section.

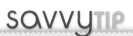
savvyTIP

Have some overripe fruits in your kitchen? Don't throw them out. Use them to make quick and healthy desserts. Freeze grapes (pulled from the stems) overnight and thaw for five minutes before eating as a snack. Freeze bananas to use in your next batch of homemade cake or muffins. Make applesauce from apples, or homemade jam with strawberries, peaches, or plums.

pie shells

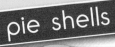

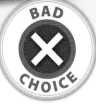

Pillsbury
9" Pie Crusts (Frozen)

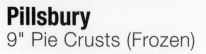

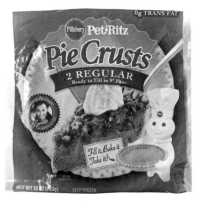

Partially hydrogenated lard *trans fat*

In Pillsbury's 9" Pie Crusts, partially hydrogenated lard (trans fat) is listed as the second ingredient. Notice that the company states this product contains a "trivial amount of trans fat" at the bottom of the ingredients list, so why does the product list "0 trans fat" on the Nutrition Facts Panel? That's because if a serving of a food contains less than a half gram of fat, the manufacturer can state that it has 0 grams of trans fat.

Sodium metabisulfite
This product contains sulfites. Buyer beware.

📖 *For more information on sulfites, refer to Chapter 3, "Worst Ingredients."*

Additives
If you are sensitive to additives, this product can push your immune system over the edge. BHA, BHT, and sulfites are known to cause various reactions. The artificial color Yellow 6 has been linked to tumors of the kidneys, and Yellow 5 may cause allergic reactions, asthma attacks, and migraines.

Nutrition Facts
Serving size 18 g

Calories 80	Calories from fat 35

Total fat 4 g
Saturated fat 1.5 g
Trans fat 0 g
Cholesterol Less than 5 mg
Sodium 70 mg
Total carbohydrates 9 g
Dietary fiber 0 g
Sugars 1 g
Protein Less than 1 g

INGREDIENTS: enriched flour bleached (wheat flour, niacin, iron, thiamine mononitrate, riboflavin, folic acid), partially hydrogenated lard with BHA and BHT added to protect flavor, water, sugar. Contains 2 percent or less of each: whey, salt, baking soda, Yellow 5 and Yellow 6, sodium metabisulfite (a preservative). Has a trivial amount of trans fats.

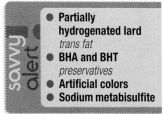

savvy alert
- **Partially hydrogenated lard** *trans fat*
- **BHA and BHT** *preservatives*
- **Artificial colors**
- **Sodium metabisulfite**

savvy tip Treats are best eaten early in the day so that you have all day to work off the extra calories. Treats eaten at night are just a recipe for weight gain.

Wholly Wholesome
Organic Traditional 9" Pie Shells (Frozen)

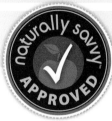

Nutrition Facts

Serving size ⅛ crust (0.88 oz/25 g)

Calories 120	Calories from fat 70

Total fat 8 g

    Saturated fat 4 g

    Trans fat 0 g

Cholesterol 0 mg

Sodium 100 mg

Total carbohydrates 10 g

    Dietary fiber 0 g

    Sugars Less than 1 g

Protein 1 g

INGREDIENTS: organic wheat flour, organic palm oil, water, organic cane sugar, sea salt.

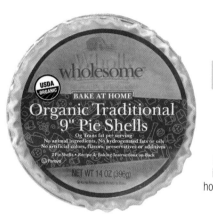

Savvy Pick

Six of Pillsbury's ingredients are red flags, including trans fats and dangerous preservatives. Wholly Wholesome pie shells are made with only five basic—and no synthetic—ingredients. That's as close to homemade as it gets.

What is ...
Organic Flour?

In order for wheat to be designated organic, third-party certifiers must ensure that it was grown without the use of synthetic fertilizers or pesticides, and farmers have to show that no chemicals have been applied to the land for three years before harvesting the grain. No toxic fumigants or other treatments can be applied to the wheat or even to other products in the storage facility during a certain time period before the organic product is stored.

cheesecake

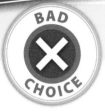

Cheesecake Factory
Berry White Chocolate Raspberry

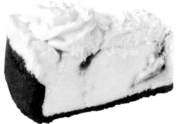

Calories
Let's keep in mind that if the average person eats 2,000 calories a day, this one piece of cake would represent over one-third of her calories and a day's worth of fat.

Never-ending ingredients list
Is this piece of cake really worth it? After analyzing the ingredients list and Nutrition Facts panel, it was unanimous: no way! Keep this one under wraps—literally. There are too many red-flag ingredients in this cake, including artificial flavors (which appear four times).

savvy alert
- **Polysorbate 80** *emulsifier*
- **High-fructose corn syrup** (HFCS)
- **Artificial flavor**
- **Artificial color**
- **Sodium benzoate** *preservative*

Nutrition Facts
Serving size 1 slice (approx. 151 g)

Calories 680 per slice	
Calories from fat 420	
Total fat 47 g	
Saturated fat 29 g	
Trans fat 1.5 g	
Cholesterol 190 mg	
Sodium 290 mg	
Total carbohydrates 61 g	
Dietary fiber 1 g	
Sugars 50 g	
Protein 8 g	

INGREDIENTS: cream cheese (pasteurized cultured milk and cream, salt, stabilizers [xanthan, carob bean, and/or guar gums]), cream (cream, carrageenan, monoglycerides and diglycerides, polysorbate 80), sugar, chocolate crumb (enriched wheat flour [wheat flour, niacin, reduced iron, thiamine mononitrate, riboflavin, folic acid], sugar, palm oil, cocoa processed with alkali, high-fructose corn syrup, corn flour, caramel color, whey [milk], salt, baking soda, soy lecithin), eggs, white pastel ribbons (sugar, palm kernel and palm oils, whey [milk], nonfat milk, soy lecithin, titanium dioxide, natural and artificial flavor), raspberry puree (fruits [raspberries, raspberry puree concentrate], sugar, corn syrup, fruit pectin, citric acid, color [anthocyanins, Red 3], natural and artificial flavor, potassium sorbate [preservative]), powdered sugar (sugar, corn starch), white ice-cap coating (sugar, fractionated palm kernel oil, whey [milk], nonfat milk powder, soy lecithin, monoglycerides, titanium dioxide, natural and artificial flavor), margarine (palm oil, water, salt, monoglycerides and diglycerides, soy lecithin, sodium benzoate [preservative], artificial flavor, beta-carotene [color], vitamin A palmitate), vanillin [artificial flavor].

calories galore

Petite Sonya Thomas holds the record for cheesecake eating: 11 pounds in only nine minutes! That's about 16,016 calories, 1,126 grams of fat in just one sitting. She claims walking on a treadmill for two hours a day helps to keep her figure in check.

Pamela's
White Chocolate Raspberry Cheesecake

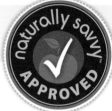

naturally savvy APPROVED

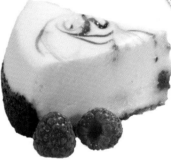

Nutrition Facts

Serving size 1 slice (94 g)

Calories 360	Calories from fat 210
Total fat 23 g	
Saturated fat 14 g	
Trans fat 0 g	
Cholesterol 110 mg	
Sodium 310 mg	
Total carbohydrates 32 g	
Dietary fiber 0.5 g	
Sugars 25 g	
Protein 6 g	

INGREDIENTS: **cheesecake:** cream cheese (pasteurized nonfat milk and milk fat, cheese culture, salt, stabilizers [xanthan and/or carob bean and/or guar gums]), organic sugar, eggs, raspberries, organic sour cream (cultured grade A pasteurized organic light cream, organic nonfat milk, microbial enzymes, live and active cultures), white chocolate (organic sugar, organic cocoa butter, organic milk powder, soy lecithin non-GMO, organic vanilla), natural vanilla. **crust:** crumb (organic evaporated cane sugar, nonhydrogenated palm oil, organic cocoa powder (contains alkali), flour base (brown rice flour, white rice flour, tapioca starch, sweet rice flour, xanthan gum), eggs, natural flavorings, grainless and aluminum-free baking powder (sodium bicarbonate, sodium acid pyrophosphate, potato starch), sea salt, xanthan gum, ammonium bicarbonate, butter.

Savvy Pick

For this comparison, Pamela's takes the cake! Both of these cheesecakes contain a lot of ingredients, but the quality of the ingredients makes Pamela's the clear winner. And if you're wondering what it tastes like, it's amazing.

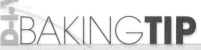

DIY BAKING**TIP**

We recommend baking with aluminum-free baking powder like Pamela does. Significant evidence suggests that regular consumption of aluminum is linked to Alzheimer's disease. Plus, we think non-aluminum baking powder tastes better, and so do pastry chefs!

brownies

BAD X **CHOICE**

Little Debbie
Fudge Brownies with English Walnuts

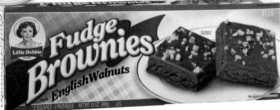

Bad all around

When you remove the trans fats, HFCS, preservatives, and artificial colors from Little Debbie Brownies, how much of the 280 calories and 12 grams of fat is made up of "real" food? We're shocked that the warnings on the package provided by this manufacturer are about wheat, nuts, soy, eggs, and almonds, when "America's Favorite" contains so many other worrisome ingredients!

Partially hydrogenated oils *trans fats*

The National Academy of Sciences has concluded that there is no safe level of trans fat consumption, as any amount will increase your risk of heart disease. One caveat: the NAS acknowledges that it is very difficult to get zero unless you adopt a vegan diet.

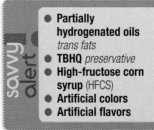

savvy alert

- **Partially hydrogenated oils** *trans fats*
- **TBHQ** *preservative*
- **High-fructose corn syrup** (HFCS)
- **Artificial colors**
- **Artificial flavors**

Nutrition Facts
Serving size 1 brownie (61 g)

Calories 280	Calories from fat 110

Total fat 12 g	
Saturated fat 3.5 g	
Trans fat 0 g	
Cholesterol 10 mg	
Sodium 150 mg	
Total carbohydrates 40 g	
Dietary fiber 1 g	
Sugars 21 g	
Protein 3 g	

INGREDIENTS: enriched bleached flour (wheat flour), niacin, reduced iron, thiamine mononitrate [vitamin B1], riboflavin [vitamin B2], folic acid), corn syrup, partially hydrogenated soybean and cottonseed oil with TBHQ to preserve flavor, sugar, dextrose, cocoa, water, high-fructose corn syrup, walnuts, eggs, soy lecithin, cornstarch, salt, colors (caramel color, Red 40), leavening (sodium aluminum phosphate, baking soda), natural and artificial flavors, whey (milk), egg whites, citric acid, sorbic acid (preservative), almonds.

savvy tip Brownies don't need to rise like other baked goods do, so it's easy to make them gluten free. Look for the many delicious gluten-free mixes on the market.

VitaBrownie
Deep & Velvety Chocolate

Nutrition Facts
Serving size 1 brownie (55 g)

Calories 100	Calories from fat 15
Total fat 2 g	
Saturated fat 0.5 g	
Trans fat 0 g	
Cholesterol 0 mg	
Sodium 120 mg	
Total carbohydrates 23 g	
Dietary fiber 6 g	
Sugars 8 g	
Protein 4 g	

NGREDIENTS: water, whole wheat flour, egg whites, maltitol, organic sugar, cocoa (processed with alkali), chocolate chips (sugar, chocolate liquor, cocoa butter), soy fiber, inulin, wheat gluten, dried honey, erythritol, wheat protein isolate, Fruitrim (grape juice, brown rice syrup), walnuts, natural flavor, leavening (potassium bicarbonate, sodium acid pyrophosphate), lecithin, sea salt, xanthan gum, vitamin A, vitamin B_6, vitamin B_{12}, vitamin C, vitamin D, vitamin E, folic acid, iron, biotin, zinc.

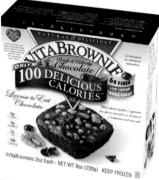

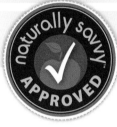

 Savvy Pick
A snack that packs 6 grams of fiber, 4 grams of protein, and only 2 grams of fat into a 100-calorie treat . . . in our opinion, VitaBrownie is the perfect snack. We wish all junk food was this healthy.

Honorable Mentions

❖ Pamela's
Chocolate Brownie Mix

❖ Whole Foods 365 Everyday Value
Chocolate Brownie Mix

❖ Vermont Brownie Company

❖ No-Pudge!
Fudge Brownie Mix

What is ...
Erythritol & Maltitol

These sugar alcohols have been approved for use by the FDA and are considered safe sugar substitutes. They have almost no calories, minimally affect blood sugar levels, and don't cause tooth decay.

cinnamon buns—refrigerated dough

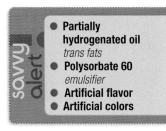

Pillsbury
Cinnamon Rolls (with Icing)

Nutrition Facts
Serving size 1 serving (44 g)

Calories With icing: 140	
Calories from fat 45	
Total fat 5 g	
Saturated fat 1.5 g	
Trans fat 2 g	
Cholesterol 0 mg	
Sodium 340 mg	
Total carbohydrates 23 g	
Dietary fiber 0.5 g	
Sugars 9 g	
Protein 2 g	

Partially hydrogenated oil *trans fat*
Prior to 2006, food manufacturers weren't required to declare trans fat on the nutrition facts panel. Since then many packaged goods companies have reformulated their recipes to remove the trans fat. We hope Pillsbury follows suit.

Sodium acid pyrophosphate
This phosphate is commonly used to prevent discoloration. Consumed in excess, phosphorous in any form can throw off your body's balance of calcium and other minerals. The sodium acid pyrophosphate in cinnamon buns won't hurt you in the least; it's the phosphorous in sodas and high meat consumption you need to watch out for.

📖 *For more details, refer to the glossary.*

savvy alert
- **Partially hydrogenated oil** *trans fats*
- **Polysorbate 60** *emulsifier*
- **Artificial flavor**
- **Artificial colors**

INGREDIENTS: enriched flour bleached (wheat flour, niacin, ferrous sulfate, thiamine mononitrate, riboflavin, folic acid), water, sugar, partially hydrogenated soybean oil, dextrose, wheat starch, baking powder (sodium acid pyrophosphate, baking soda), palm and soybean oil, whey, salt, cinnamon, cornstarch, corn syrup solids, monoglycerides and diglycerides, cellulose gum, potassium sorbate (preservative), polysorbate 60, artificial flavor, Yellow 5 and Red 40 color.

savvy tip Cinnamon and honey are known to balance blood sugar levels. When you crave something sweet, drizzle some honey over plain yogurt and sprinkle with cinnamon.

Immaculate Baking Co.
Cinnamon Rolls (with Icing)

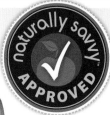

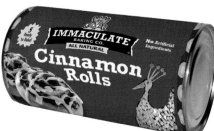

Nutrition Facts

Serving size 1 roll (99 g)

Calories With icing:	350
Without icing:	280
Calories from fat 120 for both	
Total fat 14 g	
Saturated fat 6 g	
Trans fat 0 g	
Cholesterol 0 mg	
Sodium 650 mg	
Total carbohydrates 51 g	
Dietary fiber 1 g	
Sugars 20 g	
Protein 4 g	

INGREDIENTS: **cinnamon roll:** unbleached, unbromated wheat flour (enriched with niacin, iron, thiamine mononitrate, riboflavin, folic acid), water, palm fruit oil with beta-carotene (natural color) and canola oil, sugar, leavening (sodium acid pyrophosphate, baking soda), cinnamon, potassium chloride, wheat starch, salt, cultured wheat starch, natural flavor (corn and/or soybean oil, milk), citric acid, vegetable monoglycerides and diglycerides, xanthan gum, annatto (natural color); **vanilla icing:** powdered sugar (sugar, cornstarch), sugar, water, corn syrup, canola and palm fruit oils, salt, vegetable monoglycerides and diglycerides, xanthan, locust bean and guar gums, natural flavor.

Savvy Pick

Pillsbury's serving size is less than half of Immaculate Baking Co.'s. Eat two of them and the playing field evens out for calories, fat, and sodium. But here's the real issue: is something really a treat when it contains preservatives, trans fats, polysorbate 60, and artificial colors and flavor? Immaculate Baking Co. can claim victory on this one for its much cleaner list of ingredients.

What is ... *bromated wheat flour*

Bromated flour has been treated with potassium bromate to improve dough elasticity and produce a higher-rising bread. Potassium bromate is a potential carcinogen that has been associated with thyroid dysfunction and has been banned in some countries. To avoid bromated flour, read labels carefully and choose products made with organic flour or unbromated wheat flour, as seen in the ingredients list of Immaculate Baking Co.'s Cinnamon Rolls.

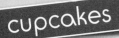

cupcakes

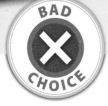

Hostess Cupcakes

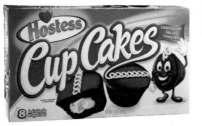

Nutrition Facts

Serving size 1 cupcake (50 g)

Calories 180	Calories from fat 50
Total fat 6 g	
Saturated fat 3 g	
Trans fat 0 g	
Cholesterol 5 mg	
Sodium 270 mg	
Total carbohydrates 30 g	
Dietary fiber Less than 1 g	
Sugars 21 g	
Protein 1 g	

High-fructose corn syrup

Bad press surrounding HFCS prompted the Corn Refiners Association to respond with a solution to repair the sweetener's reputation. The organization is currently petitioning the FDA to change HFCS on labels to more natural-sounding "corn sugar"—which sounds a lot like "cane sugar."

Misleading names

Further to the point above, other foods have successfully rebranded themselves with the FDA's approval. For instance rapeseed oil is now labeled "canola oil." Perhaps the most dangerously misleading new name to gain FDA approval is "Aminosweet": the chemical sweetener aspartame—source of countless consumer complaints—dressed in sheep's clothing.

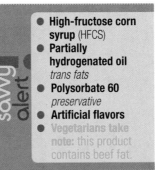

savvy alert

- **High-fructose corn syrup** (HFCS)
- **Partially hydrogenated oil** *trans fats*
- **Polysorbate 60** *preservative*
- **Artificial flavors**
- Vegetarians take note: this product contains beef fat.

INGREDIENTS: sugar, water, enriched bleached wheat flour (flour, reduced iron, ferrous sulfate, B vitamins [niacin, thiamine mononitrate (B₁), riboflavin (B₂), folic acid]), corn syrup, palm oil, high-fructose corn syrup, cocoa, partially hydrogenated vegetable and/or animal shortening (soybean cottonseed and/or animal shortening [soybean, cotton seed and/or canola oil, beef fat]). Contains 2 percent or less of modified cornstarch, glucose, whey, salt, soy protein isolate, calcium and sodium caseinate, leavenings (sodium acid pyrophosphate, baking soda, monocalcium phosphate), cocoa processed with alkali, soy lecithin, chocolate liquor, soybean oil, modified wheat starch, sodium stearate, calcium carbonate, calcium sulfate, agar, locust bean gum, dextrose, sodium phosphate, polysorbate 60, sodium stearoyl lactylate, cellulose gum, soy flour, cornstarch, monoglycerides and diglycerides, gelatin, natural and artificial flavors (contains butter), eggs, corn syrup solids, potassium sorbate and sorbic acid (preservatives).

savvy tip Many natural and organic products mentioned in this section are found in the freezer section because they don't contain the chemicals and preservatives found in many standard products, so they are not shelf stable.

Organic Pantry
Devils Delight

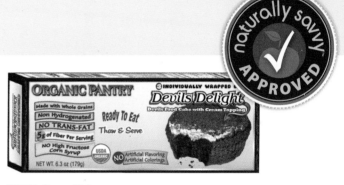

Nutrition Facts

Serving size 1 cake (60 g)

Calories 220	Calories from fat 100
Total fat 11 g	
Saturated fat 6 g	
Trans fat 0 g	
Cholesterol 45 mg	
Sodium 200 mg	
Total carbohydrates 29 g	
Dietary fiber 5 g	
Sugars 15 g	
Protein 4 g	

INGREDIENTS: organic whole wheat flour, organic sugar, organic unbleached flour (niacin, reduced iron, thiamine mononitrate [vitamin B_1], riboflavin [vitamin B_2], folic acid), organic evaporated cane juice syrup, organic unsalted butter, organic whole milk, organic palm oil shortening (sustainable source), organic whole eggs, organic inulin (Jerusalem artichoke), organic cocoa powder (alkalized), organic powdered sugar (cornstarch), organic powdered egg whites, organic vanilla extract, organic baking soda (all natural), gum acacia, xanthan gum, sea salt.

Savvy Pick:
Your first instinct might be to think twice about eating an Organic Pantry Devils Delight cupcake since each serving is higher in fat and calories than a Hostess Cupcake, but read on and you'll see that each Devils Delight cupcake has less sodium and sugar than a Hostess Cupcake, plus it has 4 grams of protein and 5 grams of fiber—both rare finds in junk food. The fiber comes from inulin, which binds to cholesterol, excess fat, and hormones (like estrogen) and removes them from the body via the stool.

Honorable Mention
❖ Shabtai *Ring Tings*

What is ...

Inulin Inulin is a type of dietary fiber that is found naturally in many foods. Food manufacturers like to extract inulin from chicory root to replace flour, fat, and sugar. Inulin is a prebiotic, so it promotes healthy gut bacteria, aids digestion, and increases calcium absorption through the intestines. It is also available in supplement form. We love Fiberrific's inulin-based fiber because it's tasteless, odorless, and has no texture, so it blends beautifully into water and baked treats.

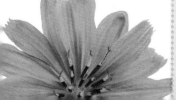

donuts

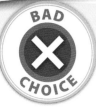

Entenmann's
Rich Frosted Donuts

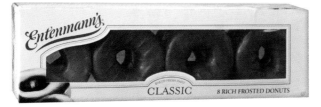

Nutrition Facts

Serving size 1 donut (60 g)

Calories 300	Calories from fat 180
Total fat 20 g	
Saturated fat 13 g	
Trans fat 0 g	
Cholesterol 10 mg	
Sodium 190 mg	
Total carbohydrates 30 g	
Dietary fiber 1 g	
Sugars 17 g	
Protein 2 g	

HFCS and mercury

Two studies have found that many products containing high-fructose corn syrup are contaminated with mercury, an extremely hazardous metal that is toxic to the nervous system.

Gums (cellulose, xanthan, karaya, guar)

Gums are safe and need not cause concern (they are derived from natural sources). Gums are added to thicken a wide range of foods. Some forms of gum are made from corn—if you have a corn allergy, double-check with the manufacturer before eating a product that contains it.

📖 *For more details on the types of gums, refer to the glossary.*

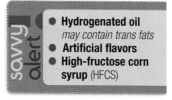

savvy alert
- **Hydrogenated oil** *may contain trans fats*
- **Artificial flavors**
- **High-fructose corn syrup** (HFCS)

INGREDIENTS: sugar, enriched wheat flour, palm oil, water, hydrogenated palm kernel oil, cocoa, soybean oil, nonfat milk, soy flour, natural and artificial flavors, egg yolks, leavening (baking soda, sodium acid pyrophosphate, sodium aluminum phosphate), high-fructose corn syrup, dextrose, salt, pregelatinized wheat starch, corn syrup, soy lecithin, monoglycerides and diglycerides, potassium sorbate (preservative), cellulose gum, guar gum, tapioca dextrin, xanthan gum, karaya gum, beta-carotene (color), caramel color.

fructooligosaccharides

A naturally occurring sugar extracted from fruits and vegetables. It helps to improve colon health by promoting the growth of good bacteria in the intestines.

Kinnikinnick
Chocolate Dipped Donuts

Nutrition Facts
Serving size 1 donut (57 g)

Calories 220	Calories from fat 50
Total fat 6 g	
Saturated fat 3 g	
Trans fat 0 g	
Cholesterol 0 mg	
Sodium 200 mg	
Total carbohydrates 41 g	
Dietary fiber 2 g	
Sugars 19 g	
Protein 2 g	

INGREDIENTS: *icing:* (sugar, water, glucose, cocoa powder), sugar, white rice flour, tapioca starch, water, whole eggs, sweet rice flour, palm fruit oil (nonhydrogenated), fructooligosaccharides (FOS), yeast, pea protein, egg whites, xanthan gum, fruit concentrate (dextrose, dextrin, fiber), salt, rice bran extract, cellulose, KinnActive baking powder, sodium acid pyrophosphate, sodium bicarbonate, pea starch, monocalcium phosphate, glucono delta-lactone, sodium bicarbonate, nutmeg.

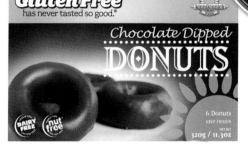

GlutenFree has never tasted so good.®

Chocolate Dipped
DONUTS

6 Donuts
KEEP FROZEN
NET WT
320g / 11.3OZ

naturally savvy APPROVED

Savvy Pick
With a lot less fat than Entenmann's donuts and free from gluten, dairy, casein, lactose, and nuts, Kinnikinnick is a donut we would even be happy to offer Homer Simpson. And that's the "hole" truth.

What is ...
Celiac Disease (CD)?

When people with this autoimmune disease ingest gluten, a protein found in grain, their body elicits an immune response that damages the villi—the absorptive surface—of the small intestine, interfering with the absorption of nutrients. The classic symptoms of CD are chronic diarrhea, abdominal bloating or pain, constipation, vomiting, and/or fatigue. Accurate testing is available, but the only treatment at this time is to completely eliminate foods containing gluten, especially wheat, barley, and rye. For more information, visit www.celiac.org.

chocolate cake mix

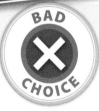

Duncan Hines Moist Deluxe
Devil's Food Cake Mix

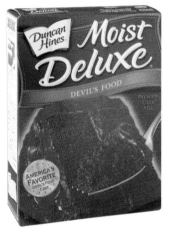

Shortening

The word *shortening* can refer to any fat that is used for baking, such as butter, lard, or margarine. Vegetable shortening is made from vegetable oils, like soybean and cottonseed oil. Since shortening blends well with flour, it is ideal for pastries and gives our baked goods a light, fluffy texture. Unfortunately, most shortening contains dangerous trans fats, including the shortening used to make Duncan Hines Devil's Food Cake Mix.

Propylene glycol

This preservative and humectant (used to retain moisture) is found in foods such as cake mixes and fat-free ice cream. Though the FDA has deemed it safe for human consumption, there have been reports of toxicity issues. Propylene glycol may be toxic to the central nervous system and even the heart.

Nutrition Facts

Serving size ½ package/12 servings per container (43 g)

Calories 170	Calories from fat 40

Total fat 4.5 g	
Saturated fat 1.5 g	
Trans fat 0 g	
Cholesterol 0 mg	
Sodium 330 mg	
Total carbohydrates 33 g	
Dietary fiber 1 g	
Sugars 19 g	
Protein 2 g	

INGREDIENTS: sugar, enriched bleached wheat flour (flour, niacin, reduced iron, thiamine mononitrate, riboflavin, folic acid), vegetable oil shortening (partially hydrogenated soybean oil, propylene glycol, monoesters and diesters of fats, monoglycerides and diglycerides), cocoa powder processed with alkali, dextrose, leavening (sodium bicarbonate, dicalcium phosphate, sodium aluminum phosphate, monocalcium phosphate). Contains 2 percent or less of each: modified food starch, wheat starch, polyglycerol esters of fatty acids, salt, cellulose gum, xanthan gum, maltodextrin, artificial flavors.

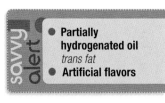

savvy alert
- **Partially hydrogenated oil** *trans fat*
- **Artificial flavors**

savvy tip Add a tablespoon of ground flaxseed or chia, some pureed fruit, a little whole grain flour, or some ground, raw nuts into your baking to up the nutritional value.

DR. OETKER
Organic Cake Mix—Chocolate

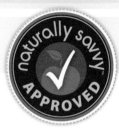

Nutrition Facts
Serving size 1/12 package/12 servings per container (40 g)

Calories 150	Calories from fat 5
Total fat 0.5 g	
Saturated fat 0 g	
Trans fat 0 g	
Cholesterol 0 mg	
Sodium 280 mg	
Total carbohydrates 32 g	
Dietary fiber 2 g	
Sugars 17 g	
Protein 2 g	

INGREDIENTS: organic enriched wheat flour (wheat flour, niacin, reduced iron, thiamine mononitrate, riboflavin, folic acid), organic cane sugar, organic cocoa, baking soda, cream of tartar, salt, organic locust bean gum.

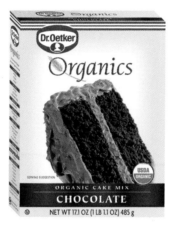

Dr. Oetker
Organics
ORGANIC CAKE MIX
CHOCOLATE
NET WT 17.1 OZ (1 LB 1.1 OZ) 485 g

USDA ORGANIC

Savvy Pick
Chocoholics everywhere are celebrating—you can have your cake and eat it too! Dr. Oetker has fewer calories and is much lower in fat than Duncan Hines, but it's the clean ingredients that make Dr. Oetker's organic mix the chocolate cake champion.

Honorable Mention
❖ Naturally Nora
Cheerful Chocolate Cake Mix

...is Flour Enriched? Why ...?

Processing flour robs it of the nutrients that exist naturally in the germ of the wheat. Since so many of us eat a large amount of processed foods (and not enough whole grains, fruits, and vegetables), flour is enriched to prevent serious nutrient deficiencies. The FDA regulates that flour must be fortified with certain amounts of B vitamins and iron.

ready-to-spread frosting

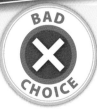

Betty Crocker
Whipped Vanilla Frosting

 Partially hydrogenated oil
trans fat

The American Heart Association recommends limiting the amount of trans fat you eat to less than 1 percent of your total daily calories. That means if you eat 2,000 calories a day, no more than 20 of those calories should come from trans fat—or less than 2 grams of trans fat a day. Most health experts recommend avoiding trans fat completely.

 Yellow 5

Why does this product need yellow dyes when the product itself is white? While Yellow 5 has not been identified as a carcinogen, it may contain carcinogenic chemicals and could cause hyperactivity or allergic reactions.

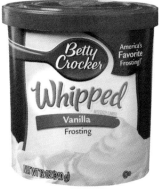

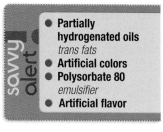

savvy alert
- **Partially hydrogenated oils**
  trans fats
- **Artificial colors**
- **Polysorbate 80**
  emulsifier
- **Artificial flavor**

Nutrition Facts
Serving size 2 tbsp (24 g)

Calories 100	Calories from fat 45
Total fat 5 g	
Saturated fat 1.5 g	
Trans fat 1.5 g	
Cholesterol 0 mg	
Sodium 25 mg	
Total carbohydrates 15 g	
Dietary fiber Less than 1 g	
Sugars 14 g	
Protein 0 g	

INGREDIENTS: sugar, partially hydrogenated soybean and cottonseed oil, water, high maltose corn syrup, cornstarch. Contains 2 percent or less of each: monoglycerides, Yellow 5 and 6 (color), salt, cellulose gel, polysorbate 80, sodium acid pyrophosphate, cellulose gum, artificial flavor, citric acid, potassium sorbate (preservative).

Cherrybrook Kitchen
Vanilla Frosting

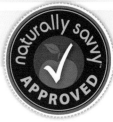

Nutrition Facts
Serving size 2 tbsp (28.35 g)

Calories 120	Calories from fat 50
Total fat 6 g	
Saturated fat 3 g	
Trans fat 0 g	
Cholesterol 0 mg	
Sodium 25 mg	
Total carbohydrates 18 g	
Dietary fiber 0 g	
Sugars 17 g	
Protein 0 g	

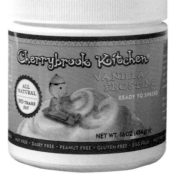

INGREDIENTS: confectionary sugar, palm oil, water, corn syrup, vegetable glycerin (derived from palm), natural vanilla flavor, salt, xanthan gum, phosphoric acid.

Savvy Pick
In comparing icing to icing, Cherrybrook Kitchen is transfat free, and is free of artificial colors, flavors and preservatives, making it the undisputed winner. As for Betty Crocker, keep the lid on this one.

Honorable Mention

❖ Naturally Nora
   frosting mixes

D-I-Y Vanilla Frosting

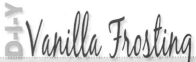

Recipe by Claire Fountain—a Naturally Savvy chef

INGREDIENTS:
- 8 tablespoons unsalted butter, softened
- 2 ounces low-fat cream cheese, softened
- 4 to 6 cups powdered sugar (confectioners' sugar)
- 4 tablespoons (1/4 cup) low-fat milk, half-and-half, or milk alternative
- 2 teaspoons pure vanilla extract

PREPARATION:
1. Cream butter and cream cheese until smooth and soft.
2. Add 3 cups powdered sugar and milk. Cream with mixer.
3. Add vanilla and blend.
4. Add remaining sugar until frosting is spreadable.

whipped dessert toppings

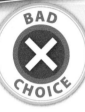
BAD ✕ CHOICE

Cool Whip
Whipped Topping

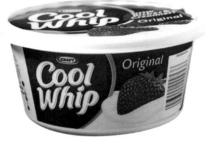

Nutrition Facts

Serving size 2 tbsp (9 g)

Calories 25	Calories from fat 15
Total fat 1.5 g	
Saturated fat 1.5 g	
Trans fat 0 g	
Cholesterol 0 mg	
Sodium 0 mg	
Total carbohydrates 2 g	
Dietary fiber 0 g	
Sugars 1 g	
Protein 0 g	

INGREDIENTS: water, hydrogenated vegetable oil (coconut and palm kernel oils), high-fructose corn syrup, corn syrup, skim milk, light cream. Contains less than 2 percent each of sodium caseinate, natural and artificial flavors, xanthan and guar gums, polysorbate 60, sorbitan monostearate, beta-carotene (color).

Sodium caseinate

This is a source of glutamate, the same dangerous ingredient known to cause reactions in those sensitive to monosodium glutamate (MSG). This is found in the natural brand too.

Nitrous oxide (N₂O)

On the label of the aerosol version of Cool Whip Whipped Topping, you will notice an ingredient called nitrous oxide. Nitrous oxide is used as a foaming agent in dairy products such as whipping cream. Animal studies have shown that it can be dangerous to the respiratory system if inhaled.

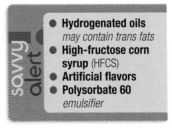

savvy alert

- **Hydrogenated oils** *may contain trans fats*
- **High-fructose corn syrup** (HFCS)
- **Artificial flavors**
- **Polysorbate 60** *emulsifier*

Trim your calories and boost your immunity by topping a bowl of antioxidant-rich fruits such as blueberries with two tablespoons of Truwhip. Still not satisfied? Drizzle a teaspoon of honey. All that goodness for less than 150 calories.

Truwhip
Whipped Topping

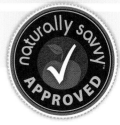

Nutrition Facts
Serving size 2 tbsp (11 g)

Calories 30	Calories from fat 20
Total fat 2 g	
Saturated fat 2 g	
Trans fat 0 g	
Cholesterol 0 mg	
Sodium 0 mg	
Total carbohydrates 3 g	
Dietary fiber 0 g	
Sugars 2 g	
Protein 0 g	

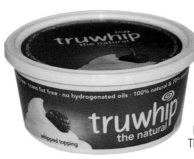

INGREDIENTS: water, organic tapioca syrup, expeller-pressed palm kernel oil, organic cane sugar, organic palm kernel oil. Contains 2 percent or less of each: organic soy protein concentrate, sodium caseinate (milk protein), organic tapioca starch, natural flavors, organic soy lecithin, xanthan gum, guar gum.

Savvy Pick
Truwhip tastes a lot like Cool Whip, but where they differ is what really counts: their ingredients. Prefer a low-fat brand of whipped topping? Then Truwhip is truly the way to go.

Honorable Mention
✦ Organic Valley
  Whipping Cream

If you choose to treat yourself to the real deal and don't mind putting forth the effort to make it, then try Organic Valley Whipping Cream. But beware: just 2 tablespoons pack 100 calories and 12 grams of fat.

What does ... Expeller-Pressed mean?

Many conventional oils are extracted using heat—which degrades the oil—and hexane, a petroleum-based solvent that is now regulated as a hazardous air pollutant. The expeller-pressing process is chemical-free and uses high pressure to get the job done without using any heat, thus protecting the quality of the oil. The result? A healthier, more eco-friendly product. Choose expeller-pressed oils whenever you have the option. They may be more expensive but are worth the extra money.

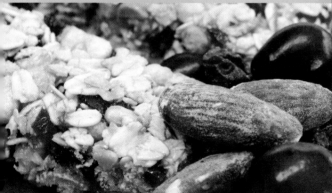

granola
bars & other
on-the-go snacks

9

- ❖ Granola bars—
  Yogurt
- ❖ Cereal bars—
  Strawberry
- ❖ Diet bars
- ❖ Toaster pastries
- ❖ Trail mix
- ❖ Yogurt-covered
  raisins
- ❖ Cheese & crackers
- ❖ Fruit leather
- ❖ Pudding cups
- ❖ Flavored gelatin—
  Ready to eat
- ❖ Beef jerky

Prepackaged Food Contains ADDITIVES

In addition to cost and waste, prepackaged foods often contain additives that may be harmful to all of us. However, additives such as artificial preservatives, colors, and flavors can especially affect a child's behavior and long-term health. While these chemicals may fall within industry standards and have FDA approval, more research is needed on the safety of many commonly used additives. It's important to read food labels carefully and to be mindful of the ingredients you put into your body.

When buying snack bars, look for those that are high in fiber, low in sugar, and free of partially hydrogenated fats.

WORST INGREDIENTS

we found in on-the-go snacks

- ⚜ Artificial colors
- ⚜ Artificial flavors
- ⚜ BHT
- ⚜ High-fructose corn syrup
- ⚜ Monosodium glutamate (MSG)
- ⚜ Partially hydrogenated oils (trans fats)
- ⚜ Sodium nitrite
- ⚜ TBHQ

also beware of

- ⚜ Annatto color
- ⚜ Caramel color
- ⚜ Carrageenan
- ⚜ DATEM
- ⚜ Propylene glycol
- ⚜ Sodium stearoyl lactylate
- ⚜ Titanium dioxide

WHY WE ♥ on-the-go snacks

Grocery store shelves are lined with ready-to-go snacks: granola bars, trail mix, yogurt cups, jerkies, and all sorts of meal replacement bars. Easy to toss into a purse or the glove compartment, they make snacking simple. Unfortunately, they can't take the place of real food, and many prepared snack foods contain unsavory ingredients such as excess (and poor-quality) sugars, artificial ingredients, and preservatives.

DON'T Be Misled

While snack bars are a great grab-and-go pick-me-up, they are just that—snacks to be eaten between meals, not as a meal. At first glance (and if you believe the advertising), snack bars appear to be packed with energizing nutrients and healthy ingredients such as fiber. The ingredients list, however, may reveal many hidden surprises, like dangerous forms of sugar, partially hydrogenated fat (trans fat), and artificial ingredients. Snack bars don't provide enough calories or nutritional value to substitute for a meal. They've been criticized for being only one step up from a candy bar, and a quick comparison proves this to be true: a standard-size chocolate bar supplies about 250 calories, mostly from sugar (20 to 35 grams) and fat (10 to 14 grams), and while granola and cereal bars typically have fewer calories and less fat, many have the same amount of sugar as a chocolate bar.

This chapter will provide you with some healthy, preservative- and chemical-free on-the-go alternatives.

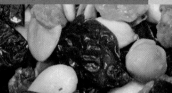

D-I-Y TIPS On-the-Go HEALTHY SNACKS

- Keep a stash of healthy dips in the refrigerator at home and at work. Top whole grain crackers with hummus, salsa, guacamole, and bean or vegetable spreads. Experiment with different vegetables such as rutabaga, daikon, parsnips, and sugar snap peas.

- Stock up on these fiber- and protein-rich snacks found at bulk food stores: dry-roasted soy nuts, chickpeas (or garbanzo beans), and green peas.

- A protein shake or fruit smoothie is a perfect, quick, and nutritious snack, especially if you don't have much of a morning appetite.

- Prepare a trail mix from dried fruit and nuts.

- Keep a protein-rich bar in your car or purse.

granola bars—yogurt

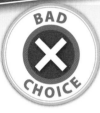

Kellogg's Nutri-Grain
Yogurt Bars—Strawberry

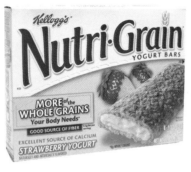

Around the World

In Britain, Kellogg's Nutri-Grain bars are made with natural colorings such as beetroot and paprika, but they contain artificial food dyes in the United States! If natural dyes are a viable option, why not go the healthier route?

Partially hydrogenated oils *trans fats*

Many people who eat bars do so in an attempt to reach a weight loss goal, but choosing a bar with partially hydrogenated oil is counterproductive. A study at Harvard Medical School revealed that a diet containing trans fat will cause more weight gain than a diet without trans fat when equal calories are consumed in both diets.

Nutrition Facts
Serving size 1 bar (37 g)

Calories 130	Calories from fat 30
Total fat 3.5 g	
Saturated fat 0.5 g	
Trans fat 0 g	
Cholesterol 0 mg	
Sodium 110 mg	
Total carbohydrates 25 g	
Dietary fiber 3 g	
Sugars 12 g	
Protein 2 g	

INGREDIENTS: whole grain oats, enriched flour (wheat flour, niacin, reduced iron, thiamin mononitrate [Vitamin B₁], riboflavin [Vitamin B₂], folic acid), whole wheat flour, high-fructose corn syrup, soybean oil (with TBHQ and citric acid for freshness), soluble corn fiber, sugar, calcium carbonate, whey, wheat bran, salt, cellulose, potassium bicarbonate, propylene glycol, mono- and diglycerides, soy lecithin, natural and artificial flavor, wheat gluten, cornstarch, niacinamide, Vitamin A palmitate, carrageenan, zinc oxide, reduced iron, guar gum, pyridoxine hydrochloride (Vitamin B₆), thiamin hydrochloride (Vitamin B₁), riboflavin (Vitamin B₂), folic acid. filling: high-fructose corn syrup, glycerin, water, fructose, modified corn starch, partially hydrogenated soybean and cottonseed oil,† nonfat yogurt powder (cultured nonfat milk; heat-treated after culturing), strawberry puree concentrate, modified tapioca starch, sugar, cornstarch, malic acid, natural and artificial flavor, cellulose gel, salt, color added, cellulose gum, DATEM, mono- and diglycerides, maltodextrin, soy lecithin, caramel color, red #40. † Less than 0.5g trans fat per serving.

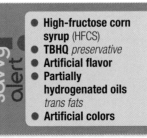

savvy alert

- **High-fructose corn syrup** (HFCS)
- **TBHQ** *preservative*
- **Artificial flavor**
- **Partially hydrogenated oils** *trans fats*
- **Artificial colors**

first comes whole grain, then comes fiber

A snack bar can be a nourishing nibble if the first ingredient listed is a whole grain, as is true of the Nature's Path bar below. Whole grains contain healthy phytonutrients, fiber, B vitamins, and minerals.

Nature's Path Organic
Yogurt Berry Strawberry Bars

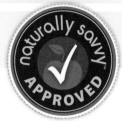

Nutrition Facts
Serving size 1 bar (35 g)

Calories 140	Calories from fat 30
Total fat 3.5 g	
Saturated fat 0.5 g	
Trans fat 0 g	
Cholesterol 0 mg	
Sodium 80 mg	
Total carbohydrates 25 g	
Dietary fiber 2 g	
Sugars 11 g	
Protein 2 g	

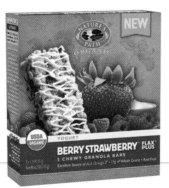

Savvy Pick

Nutri-Grain's ingredient list contains everything but the kitchen sink, including a lot of bad ingredients. Nature's Path Organic Berry Strawberry Chewy Granola Bars has a clean list of organic ingredients, so it gets our Savvy Seal of Approval™.

INGREDIENTS: organic granola (organic rolled oats, evaporated organic cane juice, organic soy oil), organic tapioca syrup, organic brown rice flour, organic invert cane syrup, organic strawberry pieces (organic strawberry juice, organic raspberry juice, organic cherry juice, organic apple puree, organic rice meal, organic soy oil, pectin, citric acid, natural flavor), organic yogurt icing (organic evaporated cane juice, organic palm kernel oil, and/or organic cocoa butter, organic cultured buttermilk powder [organic skim milk, starter culture], organic cultured nonfat dried milk [organic skim milk, starter culture], natural flavor, soy lecithin, sea salt, citric acid, organic tapioca starch), organic flaxseeds, organic acacia gum, freeze-dried organic berry blend (freeze-dried organic strawberries, freeze-dried organic raspberries), organic soy oil, evaporated organic cane juice, sea salt, natural strawberry flavor, organic molasses, citric acid.

This is a classic example of why we wrote this book...

If you just look at the Nutrition Facts panels of these two products, they appear to be almost identical. But when you take a closer look at what the products are made from, they are completely different. One is much cleaner than the other. Now that you see it for yourself, which granola bar would you choose to eat? We cannot emphasize enough the importance of reading the ingredients.

cereal bars—strawberry

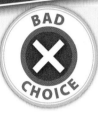

BAD
CHOICE

Kellogg's Special K
Cereal Bar—Strawberry

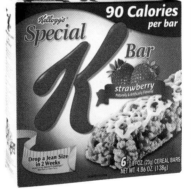

90 Calories per bar

6 (0.81 OZ. (23g) CEREAL BARS
NET WT 4.86 OZ. (138g)

Where are the strawberries?

There are no actual strawberries in this product. Instead of the beautiful real strawberries shown on the front of the box, the Special K bars give you "strawberry flavored fruit pieces" made from ingredients other than strawberries. Add some partially hydrogenated oil (trans fat), artificial flavors, TBHQ, and BHT and you get a Kellogg's Special K Strawberry Cereal Bar.

Cereal bars

Designed for people who don't have the time to sit down to eat a bowl of cereal, most commercial cereal bars are made with white flour and a jam-like filling—far from a bowl of whole grain cereal, milk, and fresh fruit. You're better off with the real thing.

Nutrition Facts
Serving size 1 bar (23 g)

Calories 90	Calories from fat 15
Total fat 1.5 g	
Saturated fat 1 g	
Trans fat 0 g	
Cholesterol 0 mg	
Sodium 85 mg	
Total carbohydrates 18 g	
Dietary fiber 3 g	
Sugars 9 g	
Protein 1 g	

savvy alert

- **TBHQ** *preservative*
- **Partially hydrogenated oil** *trans fat*
- **Artificial flavors**
- **Artificial color**
- **BHT** *preservative*

INGREDIENTS: cereal (rice, whole grain wheat, sugar, wheat bran, soluble wheat fiber, salt, malt flavoring, maltodextrin, thiamin mononitrate [Vitamin B$_1$], riboflavin [Vitamin B$_2$]), corn syrup, soluble corn fiber, fructose), strawberry flavored fruit pieces (sugar, cranberries, citric acid, natural strawberry flavor with other natural flavors, elderberry juice concentrate for color, sunflower oil), sugar, vegetable oil (soybean and palm oil with TBHQ for freshness, partially hydrogenated palm kernel oil),† maltodextrin, contains two percent or less of dextrose, sorbitol, glycerin, nonfat dry milk, natural and artificial strawberry flavor, soy lecithin, salt, natural and artificial flavor, niacinamide, color added, pyridoxine hydrochloride (Vitamin B$_6$), BHT (preservative).

†Less than 0.5g trans fat per serving.

savvy tip Most cereal bars are high in carbohydrates which quickly raise blood sugar levels. Balance blood sugar by adding protein with a handful of almonds or yogurt.

Barbara's
Multigrain Cereal Bar — Strawberry

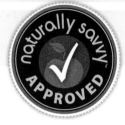

Nutrition Facts
Serving size 1 bar (37 g)

Calories 150	Calories from fat 20
Total fat 2 g	
Saturated fat 0 g	
Trans fat 0 g	
Cholesterol 0 mg	
Sodium 85 mg	
Total carbohydrates 29 g	
Dietary fiber 2 g	
Sugars 15 g	
Protein 2 g	

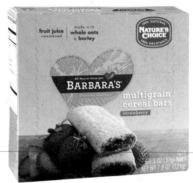

Savvy Pick
Barbara's Multigrain Cereal Bars are quite a bit larger than Special K's; however, when you even out the serving size (gram for gram), the calories and sugar are on par, but Barbara's has less fat and sodium and no trans fat, TBHQ, artificial flavors or colors. In our opinion, it's the better choice.

INGREDIENTS: **strawberry filling:** fruit juice concentrate (pineapple, peach, apple, and pear), strawberry puree, tapioca starch, apple powder, natural strawberry flavor, vegetable glycerin, locust bean gum, red cabbage and annatto (color enhancers). **crust:** pineapple juice syrup, whole oat flour, whole barley flour, whole oat flakes, rice flour, date paste, apple powder, expeller-pressed canola oil, raisin juice concentrate, malted barley extract, tapioca starch, pear powder, natural flavor, salt, aluminum-free baking powder (sodium acid pyrophosphate, corn starch, baking soda), baking soda.

Buyer Beware

Think unhealthy ingredients are only found in sweets and snacks? Think again. Carefully inspect all ingredients lists, including those on cereal boxes. You'll find high-fructose corn syrup in Kellogg's Corn Flakes, All-Bran, and Raisin Bran; Froot Loops contains trans fats and artificial colors; and BHT is added directly to cereal as well as being used in the packaging.

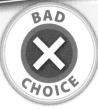

diet bars

Slim-Fast
Peanut Butter Crunch Time Snack Bar

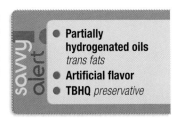

Sugar

Notice that the first two ingredients in the Slim-Fast diet bar are sugar, contributing to the 13 grams of sugar found in the product. How is this a diet bar?

Partially hydrogenated oils
trans fats

It's well known that trans fats are linked to "bad" cholesterol (LDL). But did you know that they also decrease testosterone, increase abnormal sperm, and increase the risk of low-birth-weight babies?

Vitamin-mineral blend

Although some of these terms are difficult to pronounce, they are vitamins and minerals. Specifically, calcium pantothenate is calcium, pyridoxine hydrochloride is Vitamin B_6, and cyanocobalamin is vitamin B_{12}.

📖 *See Chapter 2 for more information.*

savvy alert

- **Partially hydrogenated oils** *trans fats*
- **Artificial flavor**
- **TBHQ** *preservative*

Nutrition Facts
Serving size 1 bar (23 g)

Calories 100	Calories from fat 30
Total fat 3.5 g	
Saturated fat 1.5 g	
Trans fat 0 g	
Cholesterol 0 mg	
Sodium 70 mg	
Total carbohydrates 16 g	
Dietary fiber 0 g	
Sugars 13 g	
Protein 1 g	

INGREDIENTS: sugar, corn syrup, dry roasted peanuts, milk chocolate-flavored coating (sugar, partially hydrogenated vegetable oils [palm kernel oil, palm oil], cocoa [processed with alkali], nonfat milk, whey, salt, soy lecithin, vanillin), artificial flavor, molasses, salt, corn oil, TBHQ, and citric acid (preservatives). Vitamins and minerals: calcium carbonate, vitamin E acetate, niacinamide, folic acid, pyridoxine hydrochloride (Vitamin B_6), riboflavin, vitamin A palmitate, calcium pantothenate, cyanocobalamin (vitamin B_{12}), thiamine mononitrate.

sugar control

To reduce your sugar intake, replace sugary snacks with healthier alternatives. Some suggestions: add fresh fruit to sweeten whole grain cereals; jazz up plain yogurt with diced fresh figs, a handful of blueberries, or a teaspoon of agave.

thinkThin
Chunky Peanut Butter High Protein Bar

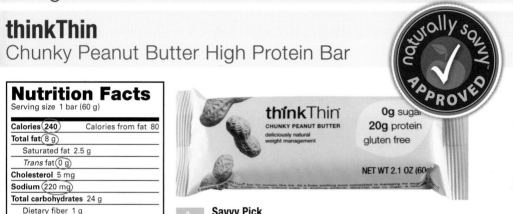

naturally savvy APPROVED

thinkThin
CHUNKY PEANUT BUTTER
deliciously natural
weight management

0g sugar
20g protein
gluten free

NET WT 2.1 OZ (60g)

Nutrition Facts

Serving size 1 bar (60 g)

Calories 240	Calories from fat 80

Total fat 8 g	
Saturated fat 2.5 g	
Trans fat 0 g	
Cholesterol 5 mg	
Sodium 220 mg	
Total carbohydrates 24 g	
Dietary fiber 1 g	
Sugars 0 g	
Protein 20 g	

INGREDIENTS: protein blend (calcium caseinate, whey protein isolate, soy protein isolate), glycerin, coating (maltitol, cocoa butter, chocolate liquor, sodium caseinate, dairy oil, soy lecithin, natural flavors, salt), glycerin, maltitol syrup, ground peanuts, soy crisps (soy protein isolate, rice flour, calcium carbonate), water, peanuts, canola oil, peanut flour, natural flavors, tricalcium phosphate, soy lecithin, salt. Vitamins and minerals: ascorbic acid, d-alpha-tocopherol, niacinamide, zinc oxide, vitamin A palmitate, electrolytic iron, calcium pantothenate, pyridoxine hydrochloride, copper gluconate, riboflavin, thiamine mononitrate, folic acid, biotin, potassium iodide, vitamin B_{12}.

Savvy Pick

"A little goes a long way" can be true in some cases, but not when it comes to trans fats. Unfortunately, the calories that come from Slim-Fast's 100 calorie bar include them. In comparison, thinkThin's 240 calories seem disproportionately higher until you consider that it is a 60 gram bar (versus Slim-Fast's 23 gram bar). You might be surprised to discover that gram for gram, Slim-Fast and thinkThin are very similar in calories and fat, although thinkThin has more sodium (which includes sodium caseinate). Another major difference: Slim-Fast has only 1 gram of protein, whereas thinkThin is actually a protein bar, providing 20 grams of protein (this helps with appetite control).

No Way, Whey!

Not just for bodybuilders anymore, whey protein provides a convenient way to introduce more protein to one's diet. Medical research has shown that the whey protein in bars and powders can significantly boost immune function, reduce cortisol production, repair tissues and muscles, balance blood sugar levels, and promote healthy skin.

toaster pastries

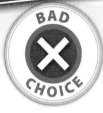

Kellogg's Pop-Tarts
Frosted Toaster Pastries—Strawberry

Misleading marketing

The statement written at the bottom of the package "Baked with Real Fruit" might give the impression that the classic frosted strawberry Pop-Tarts are at least somewhat healthy. While they are baked with real fruit such as dried strawberries, apples, and pears, they are also baked with HFCS, artificial colors, and trans fat. This is yet another example of the importance of reading beyond the front of the package.

Is this the breakfast of champions?

Starting your day (or your child's day) with a mouthful of trans fat, high-fructose corn syrup, artificial colors, preservatives, and only two grams of protein is a recipe for poor concentration, poor behavior, and poor productivity, not to mention poor health.

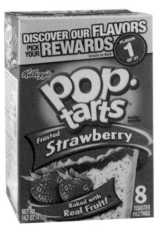

Nutrition Facts
Serving size 1 pastry (52 g)

Calories 200	Calories from fat 45
Total fat 5 g	
Saturated fat 1 g	
Trans fat 0 g	
Cholesterol 0 mg	
Sodium 169 mg	
Total carbohydrates 38 g	
Dietary fiber Less than 1 g	
Sugars 16 g	
Protein 2 g	

INGREDIENTS: enriched flour (wheat flour, niacin, reduced iron, thiamine mononitrate [vitamin B₁], riboflavin [vitamin B₂], folic acid), corn syrup, high-fructose corn syrup, dextrose, soybean and palm oil (with TBHQ for freshness), sugar. Contains 2 percent or less of each: cracker meal, wheat starch, salt, dried strawberries, dried pears, dried apples, cornstarch, leavening (baking soda, sodium acid pyrophosphate, monocalcium phosphate), citric acid, corn cereal, gelatin, soy lecithin, partially hydrogenated soybean oil,¹ caramel color, modified cornstarch, soy lecithin, xanthan gum, modified wheat starch, tricalcium phosphate, color added, turmeric color, vitamin A palmitate, Red #40, niacinamide, reduced iron, pyridoxine hydrochloride (vitamin B₆), Yellow 6, riboflavin (vitamin B₂), thiamine hydrochloride (vitamin B₁), folic acid, Blue 1.

¹Less than 0.5 g trans fat per serving.

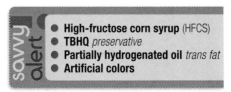

savvy alert
- **High-fructose corn syrup** (HFCS)
- **TBHQ** *preservative*
- **Partially hydrogenated oil** *trans fat*
- **Artificial colors**

savvy tip When you're buying products made with natural and/or organic ingredients, check the expiration date. Because natural products don't use artificial preservatives, they don't last as long. (Trust us, this is a good thing!)

Nature's Path Organic
Frosted Toaster Pastries—Strawberry

Nutrition Facts
Serving size 1 pastry (52 g)

Calories 210	Calories from fat 35
Total fat 4 g	
Saturated fat 2 g	
Trans fat 0 g	
Cholesterol 0 mg	
Sodium 140 mg	
Total carbohydrates 40 g	
Dietary fiber 1 g	
Sugars 19 g	
Protein 3 g	

INGREDIENTS: organic wheat flour, organic evaporated cane juice, organic evaporated cane juice invert, organic palm oil, organic apples, organic whole wheat flour, organic powdered sugar, organic cornstarch, organic vital wheat gluten, organic dextrose, organic strawberries, organic strawberry flavor, organic rice starch, sea salt, leavenings (baking soda, cream of tartar), organic tapioca starch, organic honey, organic molasses, citric acid, organic rice bran extract, betalains and paprika extract (from plants; color), organic vanilla flavor, algin, sodium citrate, monocalcium phosphate, whey protein concentrate (milk).

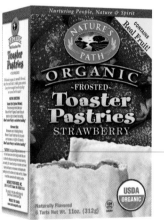

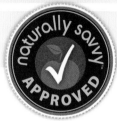

 Savvy Pick
Both of these products are on par as far as calories, fat, and taste, but Pop-Tarts' trans fat, HFCS, and artificial colors make Nature's Path the clear winner in this face-off. In fact, Pop-Tarts earns a top spot in our Hall of Shame.

What are Betalains?

Betalains are natural food colorants derived from beets.

trail mix

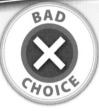

Frito-Lay
Trail Mix—Original

Partially hydrogenated oils
trans fats

Many of us would reach for a bag of trail mix over a bag of chips, thinking we are making a healthier choice, but that can be a mistake. Trans fat can lurk anywhere, and this is why it's so important to read ingredients lists. This product is one of the worst offenders in this section, containing trans fat, a major threat to our health, and artificial food coloring.

Artificial colors

Food colors actually influence how our brains perceive taste, and one study found that people rated the same food as better tasting with color added. This shows you how conditioned we are to how food "should" look, so we ignore the artificial process that is used to make it look that way.

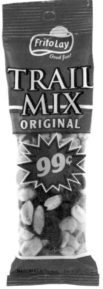

Nutrition Facts
Serving size 3 tbsp

Calories (160)	Calories from fat 80

Total fat (9 g)	
Saturated fat 2 g	
Trans fat (0 g)	
Cholesterol 0 mg	
Sodium (45 mg)	
Total carbohydrates 14 g	
Dietary fiber 2 g	
Sugars 11 g	
Protein 4 g	

INGREDIENTS: peanuts, raisins, sugar, milk chocolate (sugar, cocoa butter, chocolate liquor, whole milk powder, soy lecithin, vanilla), almonds, cashews. Contains less than 2 percent each of vegetable oil (contains one or more of the following: peanut, partially hydrogenated cottonseed and soybean, and/or sunflower seed oil), salt, artificial color (including Blue 1 lake, Blue 2 lake, Yellow 5, Yellow 5 lake, Yellow 6, Yellow 6 lake, Red 40, Red 40 lake), corn syrup, wax, dextrin, sorbitol.

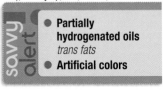

savvy alert
● **Partially hydrogenated oils**
trans fats
● **Artificial colors**

D-I-Y trail mix Combine your favorite nuts, seeds, and dried fruit (raisins, goji berries, cranberries—all sulfite-free) into a bowl and mix. Get creative with fun extras such as shredded coconut, chocolate chips or cacao nibs, mulberries, chocolate-covered peanuts, dried banana chips, or whatever else you are craving.

SunRidge Farms
All Natural Chocolate Nut Crunch

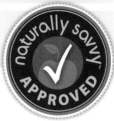

Nutrition Facts
Serving size ¼ cup (30 g)

Calories 140	Calories from fat 80
Total fat 8 g	
Saturated fat 3 g	
Trans fat 0 g	
Cholesterol 0 mg	
Sodium 15 mg	
Total carbohydrates 16 g	
Dietary fiber 2 g	
Sugars 11 g	
Protein 3 g	

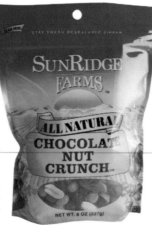

Savvy Pick
The nuts and bolts of a trail mix should include mineral-rich nuts, seeds, and dried fruit—not a mouthful of trans fats and artificial colors. And in this case both products contain chocolate for extra satisfaction. Since the amount of calories and fat are similar, we recommend SunRidge Farms. Even among its very long list of ingredients, we weren't able to identify a single red- or yellow-flag ingredient.

Honorable Mentions

✦ Bear Naked
✦ Enjoy Life (nut free)
✦ NoNuttin' (nut free)
✦ Sahale Snacks

INGREDIENTS: raisins, peanut butter chips (evaporated cane juice, fractionated palm kernel oil, partially defatted peanut flour, whey powder [milk], soy lecithin [an emulsifier]), dry roasted almonds, roasted peanuts (peanuts, peanut, canola oil and/or safflower oil, sea salt), dark chocolate chips (evaporated cane juice, unsweetened chocolate, cocoa butter, soy lecithin [an emulsifier], natural vanilla), dark chocolate stars (evaporated cane juice, unsweetened chocolate, cocoa butter, soy lecithin [an emulsifier], natural vanilla), peanut butter raisins (peanut butter coating [evaporated cane juice, fractionated palm kernel oil, partially defatted peanut flour, whey powder (milk), soy lecithin (an emulsifier)], raisins, pure food glaze), chocolate peanuts (milk chocolate coating [whole grain malted barley and corn, whole milk powder, cocoa butter, unsweetened chocolate, soy lecithin (an emulsifier), natural vanilla], roasted peanuts [peanuts: peanut, canola oil and/or safflower oil], pure food glaze), chocolate raisins (milk chocolate coating [whole grain malted barley and corn, whole milk powder, cocoa butter, unsweetened chocolate, soy lecithin (an emulsifier), natural vanilla], raisins, pure food glaze), peanut butter peanuts (peanut butter coating, evaporated cane juice, fractionated palm kernel oil, partially defatted peanut flour, whey powder [milk], soy lecithin [an emulsifier], roasted peanuts [peanuts: peanut, canola and/or safflower oil], pure food glaze).

Go Nuts for Nuts! Nuts and seeds are a good source of essential fatty acids.

yogurt-covered raisins

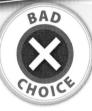

BAD ✗ **CHOICE**

Sun-Maid
Vanilla Yogurt Raisins

Partially hydrogenated oil
trans fat
Trans fat can increase bone loss, contributing to osteoporosis.

Vanillin
This is an artificial vanilla flavor made from wood pulp. Food connoisseurs notice an aftertaste after eating foods that contain vanillin. As usual, when it comes to food, there's nothing like the real thing.

Titanium dioxide
Not only is this substance found in foods, it is also an ingredient in many sunscreens. Titanium dioxide dust has been identified as a possible carcinogen by the International Agency for Research on Cancer.

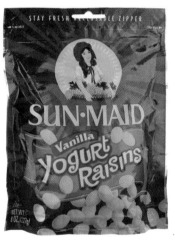

Nutrition Facts
Serving size ¼ cup (30 g)

Calories 130	Calories from fat 45

Total fat 5 g
Saturated fat 4 g
Trans fat 0 g
Cholesterol 0 mg
Sodium 20 mg
Total carbohydrates 21 g
Dietary fiber 1 g
Sugars 19 g
Protein 1 g

INGREDIENTS: raisins, sugar, partially hydrogenated palm kernel oil, nonfat milk, nonfat yogurt, whey, titanium dioxide, soy lecithin, corn syrup, vanillin, dextrin, maltodextrin, and Confectioner's Glaze.

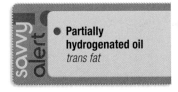

savvy alert
● **Partially hydrogenated oil**
trans fat

reasons to reach for raisins

One cup of raisins provides 1,400 milligrams of potassium—nearly a third of the daily recommended intake (DRI). Potassium works in the body to lessen the effect of salt on blood pressure and keep it in check.

SunRidge Farms
Organic Yogurt Raisins

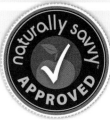

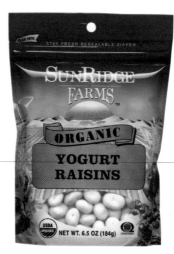

Nutrition Facts
Serving size 34 pieces (40 g)

Calories 180	Calories from fat 60

Total fat 7 g	
Saturated fat 6 g	
Trans fat 0 g	
Cholesterol 0 mg	
Sodium 25 mg	
Total carbohydrates 29 g	
Dietary fiber 1 g	
Sugars 24 g	
Protein 1 g	

INGREDIENTS: organic yogurt coating (organic evaporated cane juice, organic fractionated palm kernel oil, organic non-fat yogurt [milk], organic soy lecithin [an emulsifier], lactic acid, salt, organic vanilla), organic raisins, pure food glaze.

NET WT. 6.5 OZ (184g)

Savvy Pick
Choosing a cleaner option, when one is available, is something we always emphasize. In this case, since Sunridge Farms Yogurt Raisins are free of trans fats and are made with organic raisins, they get our Savvy thumbs-up!

Impulse buyers beware: yogurt-covered raisins are often found at the check-out line. Before you buy, read the labels carefully as they can contain partially hydrogenated oils.

Why buy? organic raisins

Almost 21 million pounds of chemical pesticides were sprayed on California wine grapes alone in 2008. Organic raisins are free of pesticides and chemical fertilizers, and are preserved naturally and without sulfites. Parents take note: it is especially important to buy organic raisins for your children, as children are highly sensitive to the toxic effects of pesticides—their smaller bodies cannot eliminate them as quickly as an adult's can. Sunview and Newman's Own Organic Raisins are two brands to look for.

cheese and crackers

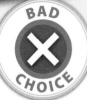

Ritz Cracker Sandwiches
with Real Cheese

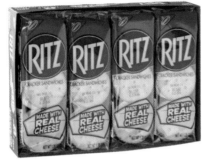

Not classy

Introduced in 1934, Ritz crackers—which are practically iconic—are popular with adults and kids alike. To our surprise, while Ritz Cracker Sandwiches do contain real cheese, they also contain three of the worst ingredients found in snack foods—trans fats, high-fructose corn syrup, and artificial colors.

Partially hydrogenated oils *trans fats*

In addition to heightening the risk of heart disease, trans fats can have a number of adverse effects on health, including promoting the onset of childhood asthma.

Peanuts

Allergic to peanuts? Take note: peanuts are listed as the last ingredient in this product.

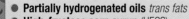

savvy alert
- **Partially hydrogenated oils** *trans fats*
- **High-fructose corn syrup** (HFCS)
- **Artificial colors**

Nutrition Facts
Serving size 39 g

Calories 200	Calories from fat 100

Total fat 12 g

Saturated fat 2.5 g

Trans fat 0 g

Cholesterol 5 mg

Sodium 460 mg

Total carbohydrates 22 g

Dietary fiber 1 g

Sugars 5 g

Protein 2 g

INGREDIENTS: enriched flour (wheat flour, niacin, reduced iron, thiamine mononitrate [vitamin B_1], riboflavin [vitamin B_2], folic acid), partially hydrogenated soybean, cottonseed and/or canola oils, whey (from milk), sugar, semisoft cheeses (made from pasteurized cultured milk, salt, enzymes), salt, high-fructose corn syrup, leavening (baking soda, calcium phosphate), buttermilk solids, sodium phosphate, natural flavor, malt syrup, soy lecithin (emulsifier), color added (contains Yellow 5 and Yellow 6), lactic acid, malted barley flour, peanuts.

savvy tip Carbohydrates should always be paired with protein, so top your plain crackers with some cheese, tuna, or peanut butter.

Late July Organic
Cheddar Cheese Sandwich Crackers

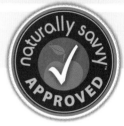

Nutrition Facts
Serving size 1 package (34 g)

Calories 140	Calories from fat 60
Total fat 7 g	
Saturated fat 2.5 g	
Trans fat 0 g	
Cholesterol Less than 5 mg	
Sodium 420 mg	
Total carbohydrates 17 g	
Dietary fiber 1 g	
Sugars 2 g	
Protein 2 g	

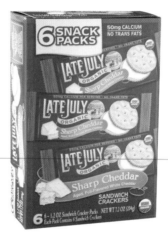

INGREDIENTS: organic wheat flour, organic cheddar cheese blend (organic cheddar cheese [organic cultured pasteurized milk, salt, enzyme], organic nonfat milk, organic whey, organic sweet cream, salt, disodium phosphate, lactic acid, enzymes, natural flavor, mixed tocopherols, organic buttermilk), organic palm oil, organic oleic safflower oil and/or organic oleic sunflower oil, organic evaporated cane juice, sea salt, leavening (baking soda, cream of tartar), soy lecithin (emulsifier).

Savvy Pick
Sorry, Ritz, but we are cracking down on bad ingredients. Late July Cheddar Cheese Sandwich Crackers are delicious and free of trans fats, HFCS, and artificial colors, making it the Naturally Savvy choice, hands down.

PICKY EATERS

Your child's food preferences may change from one day to the next. Try new foods regularly and don't be afraid to try them more than once. "Children have an abundance of taste buds so they are more sensitive to different tastes and textures, plus their taste buds are developing," says Terry Carson, Naturally Savvy's Parenting Coach. So you may have to offer new foods many times before your children develop a taste for them.

fruit leather

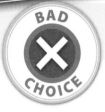

Fruit by the Foot
Strawberry

 Partially hydrogenated oils *trans fats*

They can hide where you least expect them. Who would have guessed they were hiding in fruit leathers?

Yellow 5
This is the second most widely used artificial coloring. Yellow 5 is commonly found in candy, some baked goods, and gelatin-based desserts. It is known to cause mild allergic reactions, mostly in those who are sensitive to aspirin.

Red 40—Allura Red
One study demonstrated it sped up the growth of tumors in mice, another didn't. At the end of the day, there just isn't enough evidence to guarantee its safety.

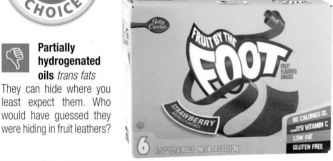

Nutrition Facts
Serving size 1 roll (21 g)

Calories 80	Calories from fat 10
Total fat 1 g	
Saturated fat 0 g	
Trans fat 0 g	
Cholesterol 0 mg	
Sodium 45 mg	
Total carbohydrates 17 g	
Dietary fiber 0 g	
Sugars 9 g	
Protein 0 g	

INGREDIENTS: pears from concentrate, sugar, maltodextrin, water, corn syrup, partially hydrogenated cottonseed oil. Contains 2 percent or less of each: carrageenan, citric acid, acetylated monoglycerides and diglycerides, sodium citrate, malic acid, xanthan gum, locust bean gum, ascorbic acid (vitamin C), potassium citrate, natural flavor, color (Yellow 5, Red 40, Blue 1).

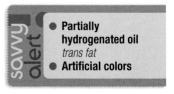

savvy alert
- **Partially hydrogenated oil** *trans fat*
- **Artificial colors**

savvy tip Try a different seasonal fruit or vegetable every time you shop for groceries. Each fruit or vegetable provides its own diverse set of nutrients. Try passion fruit, baby bok choy, lychee, blood oranges, oyster mushrooms, broccoli sprouts, and Vidalia onions.

FruitaBü
Strawberry Rolls

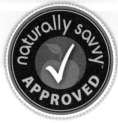

Nutrition Facts	
Serving size 1 roll (21 g)	
Calories 80	Calories from fat 10
Total fat 1.5 g	
Saturated fat 1 g	
Trans fat 0 g	
Cholesterol 0 mg	
Sodium 40 mg	
Total carbohydrates 16 g	
Dietary fiber Less than 1 g	
Sugars 14 g	
Protein 0 g	

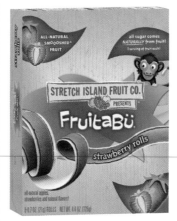

Savvy Pick
Both fruit leathers taste great, but do we really need trans fats and artificial colors by the foot? We think absolutely not. The better choice is FruitaBü.

INGREDIENTS: apple puree concentrate, apple juice concentrate, white grape juice concentrate, apple powder, strawberry puree concentrate, organic palm fruit oil, citrus pectin, natural strawberry flavor, fruit juice (color), citric acid, sodium citrate, soy lecithin.

What is... Xanthan Gum?

Often derived from corn, xanthan gum results from the fermentation of sugars by the bacteria *Xanthomonas campestris*. Xanthan gum is often added to products that have gelatinous properties, and it's also used as a thickener, stabilizer, emulsifier, and binding agent in the preparation of sauces, salad dressings, and dairy products. It is often used in gluten-free baking to replace the gluten.

pudding cups

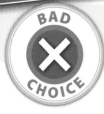

Snack Pack
Chocolate Pudding

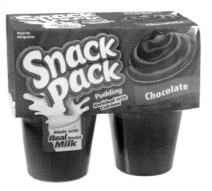

Nutrition Facts

Serving size 1 cup (99 g)

Calories 130	Calories from fat 25
Total fat 3 g	
Saturated fat 1.5 g	
Trans fat 0 g	
Cholesterol 0 mg	
Sodium 140 mg	
Total carbohydrates 23 g	
Dietary fiber Less than 1 g	
Sugars 16 g	
Protein 1 g	

INGREDIENTS: nonfat milk, water, sugar, modified corn starch, vegetable oil (contains one or more of the following: palm oil, partially hydrogenated palm oil, sunflower oil, partially hydrogenated soybean oil), cocoa (processed with alkali), less than 2% of: salt, calcium carbonate, sodium stearoyl lactylate, artificial flavors, color added.

Partially hydrogenated oils *trans fats*
An analysis conducted by researchers at the Harvard School of Public Health Department of Nutrition suggests that eliminating trans fats from our food could prevent up to one in five heart attacks and related deaths. That's a quarter of a million fewer heart attacks and related deaths each year in the United States alone.

Sodium stearoyl lactylate (SSL)
This dough strengthener is used as an emulsifier and stabilizer in puddings, icing, snack dips, and cheese substitutes. It's considered safe for ingestion, but as always, use caution when eating foods containing unnatural additives.

Refer to the glossary for more information.

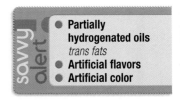

savvy alert
- **Partially hydrogenated oils** *trans fats*
- **Artificial flavors**
- **Artificial color**

savvy fact In the late nineteenth century, food manufacturers promoted puddings and custards as a sort of health food for children. Don't our twenty-first-century children wish this was true today?

Kozy Shack
Chocolate Pudding

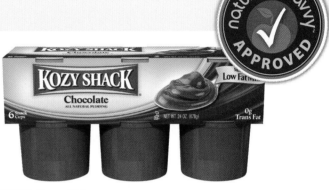

Nutrition Facts
Serving size 1 cup (4 oz)

Calories 110	Calories from fat 10
Total fat 1 g	
Saturated fat 1 g	
Trans fat 0 g	
Cholesterol 5 mg	
Sodium 110 mg	
Total carbohydrates 20 g	
Dietary fiber 4 g	
Sugars 15 g	
Protein 4 g	

INGREDIENTS: low-fat milk (including vitamins A and D), sugar, modified tapioca starch, inulin (chicory root extract), cocoa processed with alkali, salt, carrageenan, natural flavors.

Savvy Pick
The proof is in the pudding! Lower in calories, fat, sodium, and carbs, we love Kozy Shack Chocolate Pudding. It's free of trans fats and artificial ingredients, and it provides 4 grams of fiber. That's higher than most granola bars.

Honorable Mentions

✤ ZenSoy
  Chocolate Pudding (vegan option)

✤ Soyummi
  Dark Chocolate Whipped Pudding (soy)

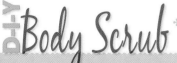

DIY Body Scrub

Can chocolate put you in the mood for the spa? Wraps, massage, and exfoliants using chocolate are the newest spa craze. Rich in antioxidants, could this be the next anti-aging trend? To create your own in-house spa experience, in a bowl combine 1 dark chocolate bar (approximately 6 melted tablespoons), half a cup of coconut oil (room temperature), 1 cup of coarse sea salt, and a few drops of natural vanilla extract. Mix until well blended. Apply the paste to your body and gently massage over your skin. Wash it off in the shower.

flavored gelatin—ready to eat

BAD ✖ **CHOICE**

Jell-O
Gelatin Snacks—Strawberry & Orange

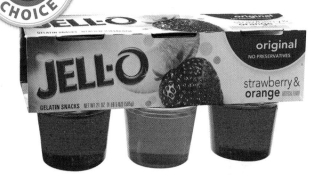

Nutrition Facts
Serving size 1 cup (99 g)

Calories 70	Calories from fat 0
Total fat 0 g	
Saturated fat 0 g	
Trans fat 0 g	
Cholesterol 0 mg	
Sodium 40 mg	
Total carbohydrates 17 g	
Dietary fiber 0 g	
Sugars 17 g	
Protein 1 g	

INGREDIENTS: water, high-fructose corn syrup, sugar, gelatin, adipic acid (for tartness), sodium citrate (controls acidity), citric acid (for tartness), artificial and natural flavors, Red 40 and Yellow 6 (color).

High-fructose corn syrup
Ingredients are listed by weight on a label. HFCS is second on this list; that means, after water, it makes up the majority of this product and it's followed by more sugar.

Gelatin
Gelatin is a protein made by boiling the skin, bones, organs, and connective tissue of animals. It may sound gross, but gelatin is really just an animal protein—not much different from the meats you eat (that is, unless you're vegetarian or vegan).

Adipic acid
Used in food to add flavor (usually a tartness) and as a gelling aid, adipic acid is considered safe for use in food, but it can be mildly toxic and is a skin irritant if handled directly.

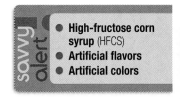

savvy alert
- **High-fructose corn syrup** (HFCS)
- **Artificial flavors**
- **Artificial colors**

veg out There are many known health benefits to following a vegetarian diet. Vegetarians have lower rates of heart disease, hypertension, diabetes, and some other cancers.

Cool Cups
Natural Orange Gels—Gelatin-free

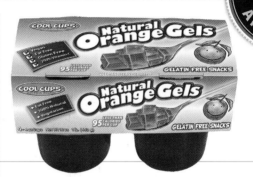

Nutrition Facts
Serving size 1 cup (113 g)

Calories 92	Calories from fat 0
Total fat 0 g	
Saturated fat 0 g	
Trans fat 0 g	
Cholesterol 0 mg	
Sodium 44 mg	
Total carbohydrates 22 g	
Dietary fiber 0 g	
Sugars 20 g	
Protein 0 g	

INGREDIENTS: filtered water, cane sugar, carrageenan, natural flavor (sodium citrate, malic acid, annatto [color], citric acid, ascorbic acid [vitamin C], vitamin E [alpha-tocopherols]).

Savvy Pick
If you're turned off by gelatin, Cool Cups are a tasty vegan option. Both products consist basically of water, sugar, a gelling agent, color, and flavor. Although Cool Cups contains two yellow-flag ingredients, in our opinion it is still the better choice since it doesn't contain HFCS or artificial colors.

Honorable Mentions
- Kozy Shack
  Smart Gels
- Simply Delish
  Jel Dessert

savvySMARTS
Think low-calorie Jell-O is better for you?

Take a look at the ingredients in Jell-O Low Calorie Gelatin Snacks, strawberry flavor: water, gelatin, adipic acid, sodium citrate, citric acid, *aspartame, acesulfame potassium,* salt, *Red 40, artificial flavor.* While keeping calories low is beneficial to overall health, artificial sweeteners, colors, and flavors do more harm than good.

beef jerky

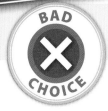

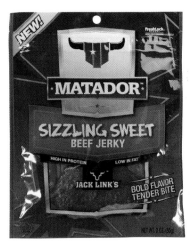

Matador
Sizzling Sweet Beef Jerky

Harmful additives
Beef jerky is a popular road trip snack, but brands that contain MSG and nitrites should be left at the side of the road.

Sodium
We like that beef jerky is rich in protein, but it's very high in sodium.

Nitrite alert
Sodium nitrite slows the spoilage of pork products and cured meats such as lunch meats, ham, hot dogs, bacon, and sausage. But nitrites combine with amines to form carcinogenic nitrosamines.

Nitrosamines
One food that almost always contains nitrosamines is bacon, due to the very high cooking temperature used to fry it. We recommend avoiding it whenever possible.

Nutrition Facts
Serving size 1 oz (28 g)

Calories 80	Calories from fat 15
Total fat 1.5 g	
Saturated fat 0.5 g	
Trans fat 0 g	
Cholesterol 25 mg	
Sodium 430 mg	
Total carbohydrates 7 g	
Dietary fiber 0 g	
Sugars 7 g	
Protein 9 g	

INGREDIENTS: beef, water, sugar. Less than 2 percent salt, fructose, flavoring, soy sauce powder (wheat, soybean, salt), monosodium glutamate, sodium erythorbate, sodium nitrite. Contains: wheat and soy.

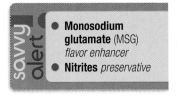

savvy alert

- **Monosodium glutamate** (MSG) *flavor enhancer*
- **Nitrites** *preservative*

beware of these ingredients commonly found in meat snacks Autolyzed yeast, BHA/BHT, MSG, large amounts of sodium, sodium benzoate, sodium erythorbate, sodium nitrite, and yeast extract.

Golden Valley Natural
Natural Beef Jerky—Original

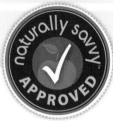

Nutrition Facts
Serving size 1 oz (28 g)

Calories 70	Calories from fat 10
Total fat 1 g	
Saturated fat 0 g	
Trans fat 0 g	
Cholesterol 10 mg	
Sodium 270 mg	
Total carbohydrates 5 g	
Dietary fiber 0 g	
Sugars 5 g	
Protein 11 g	

INGREDIENTS: beef, sugar, water, soy sauce (water, wheat, soybeans, salt), apple cider vinegar, salt, natural flavorings, paprika, natural smoke flavoring.

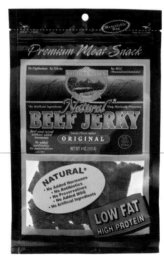

Savvy Pick

With almost a third of your day's sodium allowance, some of Matador's sodium comes from harmful additives, including MSG and sodium nitrite. Golden Valley gets our vote for being naturally seasoned and made with hormone- and antibiotic-free beef.

Honorable Mentions

❖ Shelton's
  Beef Jerky

❖ Vermont Smoke and Cure

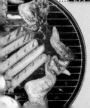

CAUTION:
Charring Meat (Barbecuing) Can Be Hazardous to Your Health

Grilling meat produces two types of potentially carcinogenic compounds: polycyclic aromatic hydrocarbons (PAHs), produced mainly in smoked foods; and heterocyclic amines (HCAs), produced mainly in food cooked at high temperatures. The following steps will reduce your exposure to PAHs and HCAs: remove all visible fat; marinate meat to prevent it from drying out; cook meat at a lower temperature than normal; and remove any burnt (black) portions on the food before eating.

candy

10

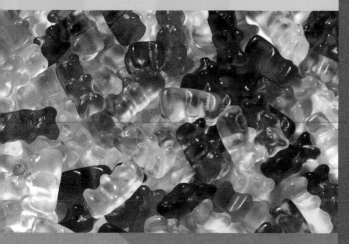

- ✣ Hard Candy
- ✣ Lollipops
- ✣ Breath mints
- ✣ Gummy bears
- ✣ Jelly beans
- ✣ Licorice—Red
- ✣ Chewing gum
  - • Bubble gum
  - • Sugar-free

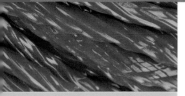

How It All Began

Candy dates back to prehistoric times, when honey was eaten straight from the beehive. The first known candy confections were fruits and nuts rolled in honey.

WHY WE ♡ *Candy* Chewy, minty, gooey, fruity, citrusy—there's a candy for everyone's taste, and we have a very big sweet tooth! Almost all Americans (97 percent) buy candy every year, and we consume about 24 pounds of candy per person. From birthdays to Halloween, it's both an everyday treat and an intrinsic part of our holidays and traditions. Not surprisingly, candy is big business. Confections ranked fourth in retail food sales in 2009, bringing in $29 billion in the United States alone.

WORST INGREDIENTS

we found in **candy**

✢ Artificial colors
✢ Artificial flavors
✢ Aspartame, sucralose, acesulfame K (artificial sweeteners)
✢ High-fructose corn syrup

also **beware** of

✢ Annatto color
✢ Caffeine
✢ Carrageenan
✢ Hydrogenated oil
✢ Potassium sorbate
✢ Titanium dioxide

CANDY SWAP

Worried about what your kids will bring home after a birthday party or a night of trick-or-treating? While it might be hard to get them to give up their candy altogether, plan ahead by stockpiling healthier options and negotiate a swap. Even better—ask them to trade their candy in for something they really want, such as a video game or a new toy.

artificial colors

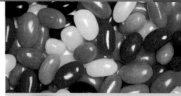

Reasons You Might Be Craving Candy

QUICK FIX

If you notice that your energy tanks about three hours after a meal, it could mean that you need a blood sugar fix. Carbohydrate-laden candy such as jelly beans and gummy bears are high on the glycemic index, and are likely to raise blood sugar levels quickly. But they're a temporary (and eventually problematic) solution to the blood sugar blues.

GUT HEALTH

A diet high in sugar promotes the growth of bad bacteria in the digestive system, which can lead to yeast problems and sugar cravings. Signs that sugar is adversely affecting your digestive system include gas, bloating, a coated white tongue, yeast infections in women, and jock itch in men (ouch).

STRESS AND FATIGUE

Are the long work hours getting to you? Feeling stressed by life causes your adrenal glands to release stress hormones, including cortisol. Instead of surrendering to your craving for sweets, candy, and other carbs, take a hot bath, get a massage, or snack on some turkey. Yup, you read that correctly: the L-tryptophan in turkey can increase your serotonin levels, which will help to counter the symptoms of stress.

MISLEADING MARKETING

Candy doesn't provide any nutritional value (there's the odd exception), but don't delude yourself into thinking that claims such as "fruit-flavored" or "sweetened with real fruit" make it any healthier than a spoonful of sugar.

Did You Know? June is National Candy Month!

savvy tip

When buying candy, read the labels. Purchase candy without artificial colors, flavors, or preservatives. Look for ingredients such as organic evaporated cane juice or other natural sugars (instead of high-fructose corn syrup), natural flavors such as real peppermint, and natural colors derived from fruits, vegetables, spices (like turmeric), and other plant sources.

Lollipop Trivia

Q: Can you name three songs with the word lollipop in them?

A:
1. "The Good Ship Lollipop" *(Shirley Temple's 1934 movie* Bright Eyes*)*
2. "Lollipop" *("Lollipop, lollipop, oh lolli-lolli-pop," The Chordettes)*
3. "Lollipop Guild" *("We represent the Lollipop Guild," Wizard of Oz)*

hard candy

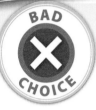

Life Savers
Hard Candy—Sugar-Free Wild Cherry

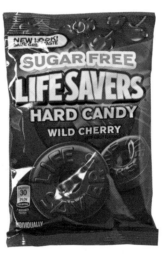

Artificial colors
Our brains are hardwired to recognize colorful food as healthy and nutritious. Artificial dyes in food and candy wake up that subconscious part of our brain to say, "I'm ripe, and I'm good for you! Eat me!"—which couldn't be further from the truth.

Nutrition Facts
Serving size 4 pieces (16 g)

Calories 30	Calories from fat 0
Total fat 0 g	
Saturated fat 0 g	
Trans fat 0 g	
Cholesterol 0 mg	
Sodium 0 mg	
Total carbohydrates 14 g	
Dietary fiber 0 g	
Sugars 0 g	
Protein 0 g	

INGREDIENTS: isomalt, citric acid, natural and artificial flavors, sucralose, Red 40, Blue 1.

Ingredients
Four of Life Savers' seven ingredients are flagged in red. This is a good example of what **not** to buy.

Isomalt
A sugar alcohol produced from beets, isomalt is typically found alongside the artificial sweetener sucralose. The combination mimics the sweetness of sugar.

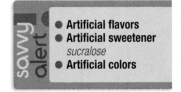

savvy alert
- Artificial flavors
- Artificial sweetener
  sucralose
- Artificial colors

Did you know? As the price of sugar decreased around the year 1700, the popularity of hard candy increased, resulting in hundreds of manufacturing facilities popping up across the United States.

Go Naturally
Organic Hard Candies — Cherry

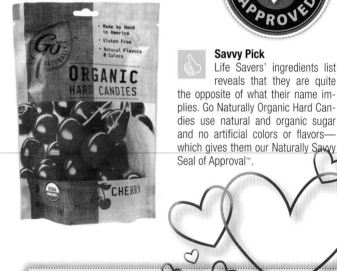

Nutrition Facts

Serving size 4 pieces (16 g)

Calories 60	Calories from fat 0
Total fat 0 g	
Saturated fat 0 g	
Trans fat 0 g	
Cholesterol 0 mg	
Sodium 20 mg	
Total carbohydrates 15 g	
Dietary fiber 0 g	
Sugars 10 g	
Protein 0 g	

INGREDIENTS: organic evaporated cane juice, organic brown rice syrup, citric acid, natural cherry flavor.

Savvy Pick

Life Savers' ingredients list reveals that they are quite the opposite of what their name implies. Go Naturally Organic Hard Candies use natural and organic sugar and no artificial colors or flavors—which gives them our Naturally Savvy Seal of Approval™.

Em♥ti♥nal Urges

We associate love, warmth, and friendship with food, especially sweets. We may "reward" ourselves with food because in our subconscious mind it makes us feel better. When we give in to emotional urges to eat, we might quickly feel better, but the effect is only temporary. The cravings will return again and again until we identify and deal with the emotions or issues we're stuffing down with food. Next time you reach for a sugary treat, ask yourself, "Do I really need this?"

lollipops

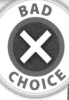

BAD ✕ **CHOICE**

Spangler Saf-T-Pops Lollipops
Assorted Flavors

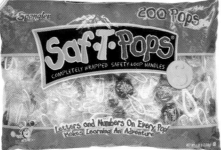

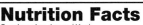

Nutrition Facts
Serving size 1 pop (11 g)

Calories 43	Calories from fat 0
Total fat 0 g	
Saturated fat 0 g	
Trans fat 0 g	
Cholesterol 0 mg	
Sodium 0 mg	
Total carbohydrates 11 g	
Dietary fiber 0 g	
Sugars 9 g	
Protein 0 g	

INGREDIENTS: sugar, corn syrup, citric acid, malic acid, artificial flavor, artificial color (includes Red 40, Yellow 6, Yellow 5, Blue 1).

Artificial flavor
Food flavors are manufactured in the same factories where perfumes are made. Fact is, the basic science behind the scent of your deodorant also determines how your candy tastes.

Artificial colors
Artificial colors give lollipops their vibrant hues. Naturally colored pops aren't nearly as bright but taste just as good.

Artificial colors
Candy makers don't have to use artificial colors—especially when natural colors approved by the FDA are readily available. Look for products that use colors from fruits, vegetables, and spices instead of artificial dyes. Examples include beet juice, paprika, and saffron.

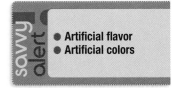

savvy alert
- **Artificial flavor**
- **Artificial colors**

did you know? The term *lolly pop* dates back to 1784. It may have derived from the word *loll* (to dangle the tongue) and *pop* (to strike or slap) for the slapping sound it would make when pulled from the mouth.

YummyEarth Organic Lollipops
Assorted Flavors

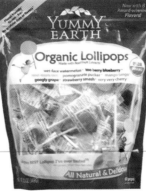

Nutrition Facts
Serving size 3 pops (17 g; 11 g for 2 pops)

Calories 70 (46 calories for 2 pops)	
Calories from fat 0	
Total fat 0 g	
Saturated fat 0 g	
Trans fat 0 g	
Cholesterol 0 mg	
Sodium 0 mg	
Total carbohydrates 17 g (11 g for 2 pops)	
Dietary fiber 0 g	
Sugars 17 g (11 g for 2 pops)	
Protein 0 g	

INGREDIENTS: organic evaporated cane juice, organic tapioca syrup and/or organic rice syrup, citric acid (from beet sugar), natural flavors, may contain organic black carrots, organic black currant, organic apple, organic carrot, organic pumpkin.

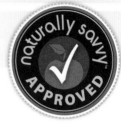

Savvy Pick
YummyEarth Organic Lollipops are made with organic sugar and without artificial food colors. Even though YummyEarth lists fruit and vegetables among its ingredients, you still need to eat five or more servings every day.

Types of natural sugar

Natural products are more likely to include fewer forms of **processed** sugar. Some natural sugars include:

Blackstrap Molasses
The thrice-boiled juice of the sugarcane plant. It contains significant amounts of minerals including calcium, magnesium, potassium, and iron.

Sucanat
(**Su**gar**Ca**ne **Nat**ural). Made from dehydrated sugar cane juice, it retains most of the nutrients of the sugarcane plant.

Brown rice syrup
A liquid sweetener made from fermented rice, it is less sweet than sugar.

📖 *Check out the glossary for a full list of alternate forms of sugar.*

breath mints

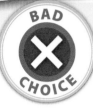

Tic Tac
Wintergreen

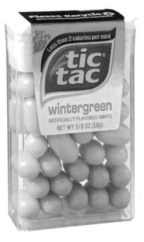

Nutrition Facts
Serving size 1 piece

Calories 1.9	Calories from fat 0
Total fat 0 g	
Saturated fat 0 g	
Trans fat 0 g	
Cholesterol 0 mg	
Sodium 0 mg	
Total carbohydrates 0 g	
Dietary fiber 0 g	
Sugars 0 g	
Protein 0 g	

INGREDIENTS: sugar, maltodextrin, rice starch, gum arabic, artificial flavors, magnesium stearate, Red 40, carnauba wax.

 Artificial ingredients
It may not seem like a big deal to have artificial flavors and color in one tiny Tic Tac, but every little bit counts—especially if you are sensitive to chemical ingredients.

 Carnauba wax
This is a natural vegetable wax used to coat candy and gum. It is considered safe for ingestion.

 Magnesium stearate
Most commonly found in pills and supplements, magnesium stearate is used as a binder and to prevent clumping. It is considered safe to ingest.

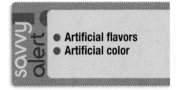
savvy alert
● Artificial flavors
● Artificial color

did you know? The menthol in peppermint stimulates nerves that sense cold in your mouth, creating the cooling sensation mints are known for.

St. Claire's Organics
Wintermints

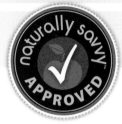

Nutrition Facts
Serving size 2 pieces

Calories 6	Calories from fat 0
Total fat 0 g	
Saturated fat 0 g	
Trans fat 0 g	
Cholesterol 0 mg	
Sodium 0 mg	
Total carbohydrates 1.5 g	
Dietary fiber 0 g	
Sugars 1.5 g	
Protein 0 g	

INGREDIENTS: organic molasses granules, organic evaporated cane juice, natural wintergreen flavor.

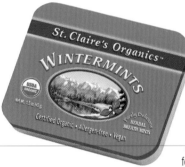

Savvy Pick
There isn't a trace of mint, menthol, or peppermint in Tic Tac Wintergreen mints. At least Tic Tac is up front about it, with "artificially flavored mints" clearly displayed on the front of the package. We pick St. Claire's for this comparison.

Honorable Mention

❖ VerMints
All-Natural Breath Mints

Good News for the Mint Family

Rosmarinic acid, a polyphenol antioxidant found in mint plants, rosemary, thyme, oregano, basil, and other herbs, has been shown to have anti-inflammatory and antimicrobial properties. What's more, animal studies using mice have demonstrated benefits for asthma, rheumatoid arthritis, and peptic ulcers, and rosmarinic acid is currently being studied for its effects on Alzheimer's disease as well.

gummy bears

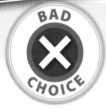

BAD **X** **CHOICE**

Black Forest
Gummy Bears—Mixed

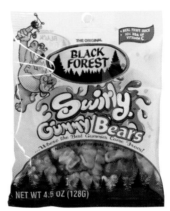

THE ORIGINAL
BLACK FOREST

Swirly
Gummy Bears
Where the Best Gummies Come From!

NET WT 4.5 OZ (128G)

Nutrition Facts
Serving size 15 pieces (39 g)

Calories 130	Calories from fat 0
Total fat 0 g	
Saturated fat 0 g	
Trans fat 0 g	
Cholesterol 0 mg	
Sodium 15 mg	
Total carbohydrates 31 g	
Dietary fiber 0 g	
Sugars 18 g	
Protein 3 g	

INGREDIENTS: corn syrup, sucrose, gelatin, citric acid, apple grape juice concentrate, sodium citrate, coconut oil, natural and artificial flavors, carnauba wax, Red 40, Yellow 5, Blue 1.

Point-of-sale homework
Gummy bears are a popular product found at the check-out counter. Next time you're waiting in line at the cash register, pick up a few bags of candy and read the ingredients. Now that you're equipped with the right information, you can make better choices.

Artificial flavors
How do artificial flavors work? Anything you can taste or smell contains chemicals that activate our sense receptors. Natural flavors are usually very complex, but as it turns out, many fruit flavors contain just a few dominant chemical components that activate our taste and smell signals. Many of these are called esters, and they can be created in a lab and added to products to give them a specific flavor. But they never taste quite like the real thing, since it would be impossible to replicate the complex flavors of real food.

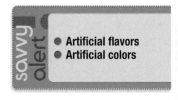

savvy alert
● Artificial flavors
● Artificial colors

savvy tip Ninety percent of tooth decay occurs within ten minutes of eating sugary or acidic foods. Drink water while or immediately after you eat candy to neutralize the acids.

Surf Sweets
Gummy Bears—Mixed

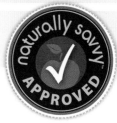

Nutrition Facts
Serving size 16 pieces (40 g)

Calories 130	Calories from fat 0
Total fat 0 g	
Saturated fat 0 g	
Trans fat 0 g	
Cholesterol 0 mg	
Sodium 15 mg	
Total carbohydrates 30 g	
Dietary fiber 0 g	
Sugars 19 g	
Protein 3 g	

INGREDIENTS: organic tapioca syrup, organic evaporated cane juice, gelatin, organic grape juice concentrate, citric acid, lactic acid, ascorbic acid, colors added (including black carrot juice concentrate, turmeric, annatto), natural flavors, organic sunflower oil, carnauba wax.

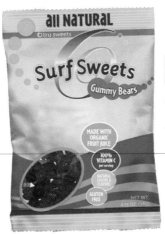

Savvy Pick

Black Forest and Surf Sweets gummy bears contain similar basic ingredients, but Surf Sweets Gummy Bears uses mostly natural rather than artificial colors. Bonus: they provide 100 percent of your recommended daily vitamin C intake per serving. For this we give it two thumbs-up.

Honorable Mention

❖ Seitenbacher Gummi Candy
   (gluten free, vegetarian, vegan)

Why ...

Gelatin Gummy bears, marshmallows, and some other candies contain gelatin that is derived from animal collagen, a protein found in skin and bones. Kosher gelatin, for example, is made from fish bones. If you are vegetarian or vegan, look for ingredients such as agar, pectin, starch, and gum arabic instead.

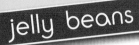
jelly beans

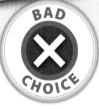
BAD CHOICE

Jelly Belly
The Original Gourmet Jelly Bean — 30 Flavors

Hydrogenated oils
If a label states "fully hydrogenated," the product is trans-fat free. If it simply states "hydrogenated," there is a chance it can contain trans fats because sometimes the terms hydrogenated and partially hydrogenated are used interchangeably.

Artificial colors
Concerns about food coloring and its link to ADD prompted European candy companies to swap blue food coloring with spirulina, a blue-green algae common to health food store shelves but not to candy. Wouldn't it be great if US food manufacturers followed their lead?

Caffeine
There is a surprising ingredient in some flavors of Jelly Belly jelly beans—caffeine. Coffee is also listed among the ingredients. If you are sensitive to coffee and/or caffeine you might want to skip these, as the smallest amount can have an effect.

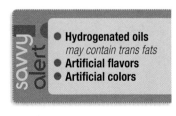

Nutrition Facts
Serving size 35 pieces (40 g)

Calories 140	Calories from fat 0
Total fat 0 g	
Saturated fat 0 g	
Trans fat 0 g	
Cholesterol 0 mg	
Sodium 15 mg	
Total carbohydrates 37 g	
Dietary fiber 0 g	
Sugars 28 g	
Protein 0 g	

INGREDIENTS: sugar, corn syrup, modified food starch. Contains 2 percent or less of each: grape juice concentrate, peach juice concentrate, black berry puree, strawberry puree, blueberry puree, raspberry puree, orange juice concentrate, strawberry juice concentrate, apple juice concentrate, hydrogenated canola and cottonseed oil, banana puree, plum juice concentrate, chocolate liquor, cocoa butter, soy lecithin (emulsifier), coconut, lemon puree, pear juice concentrate, kiwi juice concentrate, mango puree, mango juice concentrate, strawberry powder, citric acid, lactic acid, fumaric acid, malic acid, phosphoric acid, sodium lactate, sodium citrate, cocoa powder, natural and artificial flavors, coffee, Red 40 lake, Yellow 5 and 6 lake, Blue 1 and 2 lake, Yellow 5 and 6, Red 40, Blue 1 (color), tapioca dextrin, vanilla beans, beeswax, carnauba wax, confectioners' glaze, salt, caffeine.

savvy alert
● **Hydrogenated oils**
   may contain trans fats
● **Artificial flavors**
● **Artificial colors**

candy vs fruit sugar

Why is it better to get your sugar from an apple rather than from candy? Fruit comes prepackaged with nutrients and fiber that slow down your body's absorption of sugar and keep your blood sugar balanced.

SunRidge Farms
Organic Jolly Beans

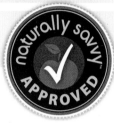

Nutrition Facts

Serving size 31 pieces (40 g)

Calories 140	Calories from fat 0
Total fat 0 g	
Saturated fat 0 g	
Trans fat 0 g	
Cholesterol 0 mg	
Sodium 35 mg	
Total carbohydrates 34 g	
Dietary fiber 0 g	
Sugars 29 g	
Protein 0 g	

INGREDIENTS: organic evaporated cane juice, organic tapioca syrup, organic grape juice concentrate, pectin, citric acid, ascorbic acid, colors added (including black carrot juice concentrate, annatto, turmeric), natural flavors, confectioner's glaze, carnauba wax, organic sunflower oil.

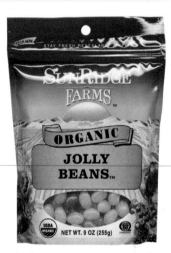

Savvy Pick

Jelly Belly's ingredients look great until we reach the artificial flavors, and then it's all downhill from there. Both products have the same serving size and calories, and both are fat free. While SunRidge Farms' Jolly Beans have double the sodium, 35 mg per serving is still considered very low-sodium by the FDA, so it isn't anything to worry about.

Honorable Mention

❖ Jelly Belly
   All-Natural Jelly Beans

Wax On, Wax Off

Food-grade waxes are safe to eat and often found in candy and chocolate. They are derived from natural sources and some have been used since the 1920s. Carnauba wax comes from the leaves of the Brazilian palm tree, candelilla wax is from the leaves of a small reed-like desert shrub native to northern Mexico, and food-grade shellac is derived from the secretion of the lac bug found in India and Thailand.

licorice—red

BAD ✗ CHOICE

Twizzlers
Licorice Twists—Strawberry

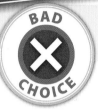

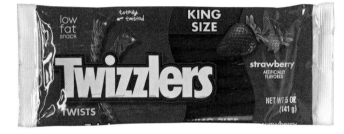

Nutrition Facts
Serving size 4 pieces (45 g)

Calories 120	Calories from fat 5
Total fat 0 g	
Saturated fat 0 g	
Trans fat 0 g	
Cholesterol 0 mg	
Sodium 80 mg	
Total carbohydrates 29 g	
Dietary fiber 0 g	
Sugars 15 g	
Protein 1 g	

INGREDIENTS: corn syrup, wheat flour, sugar, cornstarch. Contains 2% or less of each of: palm oil, glycerin, salt, artificial flavor, mono and diglycerides, citric acid, potassium sorbate (preservative), Red 40 (color), sulfur dioxide, soy lecithin.

Artificial flavor
"Artificially flavored" is usually written on the front of the package of many products that contain artificial flavors, like Twizzlers. That's a clear sign to leave it on the shelf.

Artificial flavor
So who makes all of these artificial flavors, anyway? The official job title is flavorist. Most flavorists are chemists, and they build flavors based on research that has broken down 80 percent to 90 percent of the components in most of the common flavors. Flavorists have to be creative, especially when creating tastes that don't exactly have a specific recipe—like fruit punch, which is made up of many different flavors.

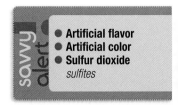

savvy alert
- **Artificial flavor**
- **Artificial color**
- **Sulfur dioxide**
  sulfites

what is DGL?

Deglycyrrhizinated licorice (pronounced: *dee-gliss-er-ize-in-ayt-ed*), or DGL, is an herbal supplement made from licorice and is used to treat gastric and duodenal ulcers. Consult your health care practitioner before trying DGL.

Newman's Own Organics
Licorice Twists— Strawberry

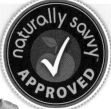

Nutrition Facts
Serving size 5 pieces (42 g)

Calories 130	Calories from fat 5
Total fat 0.5 g	
Saturated fat 0 g	
Trans fat 0 g	
Cholesterol 0 mg	
Sodium 5 mg	
Total carbohydrates 32 g	
Dietary fiber 2 g	
Sugars 10 g	
Protein 2 g	

INGREDIENTS: organic wheat flour, organic sugar, corn syrup, organic tapioca syrup, vegetable glycerin, sunflower oil, citric acid, natural flavor, strawberry juice concentrate, elderberry extract, licorice root extract.

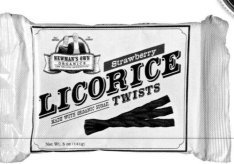

Savvy Pick

Twizzlers and Newman's Own licorice are similar in texture, taste, and calories; the only significant difference between them is their ingredients. Twizzlers' artificial flavor and color pales in comparison to Newman's Own Organics' ingredients, which include strawberry juice concentrate, elderberry extract, and licorice root extract (that's real licorice).

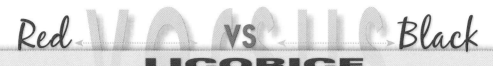

Red **VS** *Black*

LICORICE

Red licorice is made from flavorings such as strawberry, cherry, raspberry, or cinnamon. Black licorice is flavored with the extract of the root of the licorice plant. Natural brands of red and black licorice you might like to try include: Panda All Natural Licorice; RJ's Soft Eating Licorice (similar in texture to a gummy); Natural Vines Licorice; and Candy Tree Organic Twists (gluten free; available at Whole Foods Market).

chewing gum—bubble gum

BAD
X
CHOICE

Bazooka
Bubble Gum

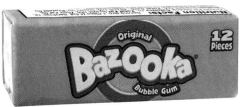

Nutrition Facts
Serving size 1 piece (8 g)

Total calories 25	Calories from fat 0
Total fat 0 g	
Saturated fat 0 g	
Trans fat 0 g	
Cholesterol 0 mg	
Sodium 0 mg	
Total carbohydrates 5 g	
Dietary fiber 0 g	
Sugars 5 g	
Protein 0 g	

INGREDIENTS: sugar, gum base, corn syrup. Contains less than 2 percent each of glycerol, natural and artificial flavors, soy lecithin, acesulfame K, aspartame, Red 40 lake (color), BHT (preservative).

Bad ingredients
We're pretty sure Bazooka Joe would be bummed to find so many unsafe ingredients in Bazooka Bubble Gum—a product marketed to children.

Artificial sweeteners
They extend how long a chewing gum's flavor lasts in your mouth, but they have potentially dangerous side effects.

Acesulfame K
Many disturbing studies of acesulfame K (K is the chemical symbol for potassium) indicate that it is no safer than aspartame.

Gum base
The formula for gum base, the main component of chewing gum, usually includes elastomers, waxes, and resins, but the ingredients can vary depending on the type of gum: bubble gum, chewing gum, or functional gum (such as medicinal chewing gum).

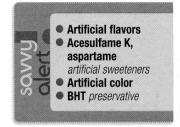

savvy alert

- **Artificial flavors**
- **Acesulfame K, aspartame**
  artificial sweeteners
- **Artificial color**
- **BHT** *preservative*

a gummy situation Chewing stimulates digestion by telling your stomach and the rest of your digestive system that food is en route, so chewing gum is a great way to stimulate your appetite. Keep in mind that chewing between meals can actually make you feel hungry.

Glee Gum
Bubblegum Flavor

Nutrition Facts
Serving size 2 pieces (2.5 g)

Total calories 5	Calories from fat 0
Total fat 0 g	
Saturated fat 0 g	
Trans fat 0 g	
Cholesterol 0 mg	
Sodium 0 mg	
Total carbohydrates 2 g	
Dietary fiber 0 g	
Sugars 2 g	
Protein 0 g	

INGREDIENTS: cane sugar, glucose, gum base (contains natural chiclé), rice syrup, natural flavors, gum arabic, resinous glaze, beeswax, carnauba wax, red beet (color).

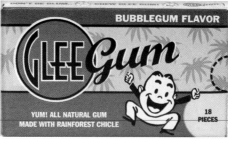

Savvy Pick
Glee offers a refreshing reprieve from unsafe synthetic ingredients, and its gum base contains chiclé—the original and natural form of gum. We just wish its flavor would last a little longer, but it is to be expected when artificial sweeteners are not used.

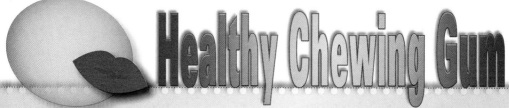

Healthy Chewing Gum

Functional chewing gum is a current trend. There's a gum for almost everything: oral health, smoking cessation, weight loss, insomnia, depression, and even for breast enhancement. Since the active ingredient is released gradually over time, chewing gum is a perfect medium for some health-promoting ingredients, such as herbs.

chewing gum—sugar-free

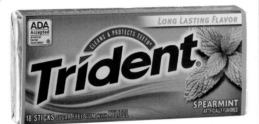

Trident
Spearmint

Nutrition Facts

Serving size 1 piece (1.7 g)

Total calories 5	Calories from fat 0
Total fat 0 g	
Saturated fat 0 g	
Trans fat 0 g	
Cholesterol 0 mg	
Sodium 0 mg	
Total carbohydrates 1 g	
Dietary fiber 0 g	
Sugars 0 g	
Protein 0 g	

INGREDIENTS: sorbitol, gum base, xylitol, glycerin, natural and artificial flavors, mannitol. Contains less than 2 percent each of acesulfame potassium, aspartame, BHT (preservative), Blue 1 lake, soy lecithin, sucralose, Yellow 5 lake. Phenylketonurics: Contains phenylalanine.

Sweet enough for you?

Trident Spearmint gum isn't just sweetened with xylitol, as indicated on the front of the package. It also contains aspartame, acesulfame potassium (ace K), sucralose (Splenda), mannitol, and glycerin.

What is phenylalanine?

One of two amino acids used to make aspartame (the other being aspartic acid), phenylalanine is an excitotoxin, meaning that it excites the neurons in the brain, and thus can worsen symptoms of ADD/ADHD and other behavioral problems.

BHT

This preservative is found in all sorts of packaged foods, but current research is looking at its potentially damaging effects on genetic material and red blood cells.

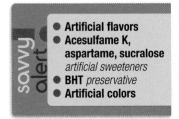

savvy alert

- Artificial flavors
- Acesulfame K, aspartame, sucralose *artificial sweeteners*
- BHT *preservative*
- Artificial colors

chew with caution

If you have mercury fillings (the silver ones), studies have shown that gum chewing can cause mercury vapors—a toxic gas—to be released into your mouth and bloodstream. Mercury exposure has been linked to multiple sclerosis, infertility, and heart disease.

Xylichew
Sugar Free Chewing Gum—Spearmint

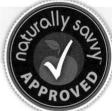

Nutrition Facts
Serving size 2 pieces

Total calories 3.8	Calories from fat 0
Total fat 0 g	
Saturated fat 0 g	
Trans fat 0 g	
Cholesterol 0 mg	
Sodium 0 mg	
Total carbohydrates 1.6 g	
Dietary fiber 0 g	
Sugars 0 g	
Protein 0 g	

INGREDIENTS: sweeteners (xylitol 70 percent weight), gum base (natural latex from sapodilla tree), natural flavor, gum arabic, lecithin, glycerin, beeswax, carnauba wax.

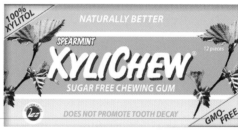

Savvy Pick
Trident may be accepted by the American Dental Association (ADA) to help prevent cavities, but its long list of red-flag ingredients can create a host of other health issues. Instead of dangerous artificial sweeteners, Xylichew is sweetened with xylitol, one of the safest alternative sweeteners based on the studies to date.

Honorable Mention
❖ Peelu Xylitol
  Dental Chewing Gum

What is ... Xylitol

Xylitol, a low-calorie sugar made from birch bark, is also produced naturally in our bodies. We make up to 15 grams of it daily during normal metabolism. The *Journal of the American Dental Association* recently reported that the sweetener "is an effective preventive agent against dental caries." Chewing the right gum really can be good for your teeth.

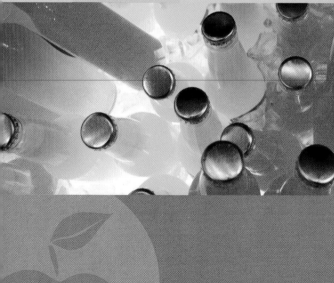

soda &
other drinks

❖ Soft Drinks
 • Cola
 • Diet cola
 • Citrus soda
 • Ginger ale
 • Iced tea
 • Lemonade
 • Orange drink

❖ Mixes
 • Single serve drink mix—Cherry
 • Low-calorie drinks

❖ Functional Beverages
 • Vitamin-enriched water

❖ Sports drinks

WHY WE *Beverages*

We love all sorts of beverages. To put this into perspective, we love coffee so much that it's the second most valuable trading commodity in the world (after oil). While some of the drinks we buy are not the best for our health, we love them anyway. But there are healthier options that will keep you sipping without overdosing on sugar, chemicals, or stimulants.

Best Hydrating Fluids

- Water: The human body is about 60 percent water—not soda, juice, or beer—and it must be continuously replenished.
- Fresh pressed vegetable juices.
- Fresh squeezed fruit juices.
- Tea (green tea or herbal teas are best).
- Organic milk (as long as you aren't allergic or intolerant to it).

WORST INGREDIENTS

we found in **beverages**

- Sugar, sugar, and more sugar, especially high-fructose corn syrup
- Artificial colors
- Artificial sweeteners such as acesulfame potassium, aspartame, Neotame, and sucralose
- Sodium benzoate and potassium benzoate

also **beware** of

- Caffeine
- Calcium disodium EDTA
- Caramel color
- Potassium sorbate
- Sodium hexametaphosphate

Bottled Vegetable Juice *vs.* Eating Vegetables

Most bottled vegetable juices are made with a blend of concentrates from tomato, carrot, celery, beet, parsley, spinach, and other vegetables. A glass of store-bought vegetable juice is a convenient and refreshing way to get some antioxidants (and often a lot of sodium), but nutritionally speaking, you're better off stopping at a juice bar for a fresh pressed veggie juice or enjoying a colorful salad.

Reasons You Might Be Craving . . . *Soda*

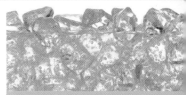

SUGAR

Cravings for sugar always have underlying causes, such as blood sugar imbalances, and sugary drinks like soda and juice perpetuate these problems.

LOW ENERGY

A can of liquid sugar provides a surge of energy. The repercussions of this bad habit, however, are dangerous and don't address the issue of why you're tired in the first place.

> *Craving soda is usually a craving for sugar, caffeine, or aspartame in disguise.*

CAFFEINE

This addictive substance is found in coffee, tea, soda, and energy drinks.

ASPARTAME

Those addicted to diet sodas are more likely addicted to aspartame's stimulating effect on the nervous system than to the taste, but more research is needed to confirm this theory.

SODA POP OR LIQUID CANDY

Soda is liquid candy. It's the largest source of refined sugar in our diet, with roughly 8 teaspoons of sugar per can. Obesity rates have risen in tandem with sugar consumption, of which soda is a main contributor. Diet soda is no better because it contains artificial sweeteners.

DRINK YOUR NUTRIENTS

An effective way to up your nutrient intake is to include green drinks and live juices in your diet. Fans report that they help to increase energy and enhance mood, memory, and sleep. Bonus: some nutrients are better absorbed by the body as fluids than from food.

Green drinks: Nutrient-rich concentrates of grasses and green vegetables, green drinks provide enzymes, antioxidants, herbs, and other ingredients in a chlorophyll-rich powdered base. They are considered a "salad in a glass." Simply mix the powder with water and drink up. Some of our favorite brands include: Barlean's, Vega, Go Greens, and Amazing Grass.

Live juices: A juice made from raw vegetables and/or fruit is considered "live" if consumed within twenty minutes of its preparation, while its enzymes are still active. Juicing is a delicious and convenient way to provide nutrients, including vitamins and minerals.

cola

BAD ✗ **CHOICE**

Coca-Cola Classic

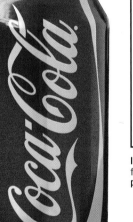

Nutrition Facts
Serving size 1 can (12 fl oz)

Calories 140	Calories from fat 0
Total fat 0 g	
Saturated fat 0 g	
Trans fat 0 g	
Cholesterol 0 mg	
Sodium 45 mg	
Total carbohydrates 39 g	
Dietary fiber 0 g	
Sugars 39 g	
Protein 0 g	

INGREDIENTS: carbonated water, high-fructose corn syrup, caramel color, phosphoric acid, natural flavors, and caffeine.

High-fructose corn syrup
In the United States, high-fructose corn syrup is the type of sugar primarily used to sweeten beverages, including soft drinks.

High-fructose corn syrup
Food and beverage manufacturers began switching their sweeteners from sucrose (table sugar) to corn syrup in the 1980s, when they discovered that high-fructose corn syrup was cheaper to make and about 40 percent sweeter.

Caffeine
A can of Coke contains 34 mg of caffeine—that's about a third of the caffeine in a cup of coffee.

Caffeine
The diuretic effect of caffeine causes the body to excrete important minerals and vitamins such as potassium, magnesium, zinc, B vitamins, and vitamin C.

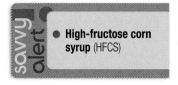

savvy alert
● **High-fructose corn syrup** (HFCS)

exercise equivalents

To burn off a cola's 140 calories, you would have to participate in one of these activities:
• 59 minutes - vacuuming • 32 minutes - washing the car • 15 minutes - climbing stairs.

Blue Sky Beverage Cola

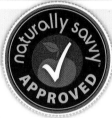

Nutrition Facts

Serving size 1 can (12 fl oz/354 ml)

Calories 140	Calories from fat 0
Total fat 0 g	
Saturated fat 0 g	
Trans fat 0 g	
Cholesterol 0 mg	
Sodium 0 mg	
Total carbohydrates 37 g	
Dietary fiber 0 g	
Sugars 37 g	
Protein 0 g	

INGREDIENTS: pure triple-filtered carbonated water, sugar, natural caramel color, citric acid, tartaric acid, natural flavors with extracts of kola nuts.

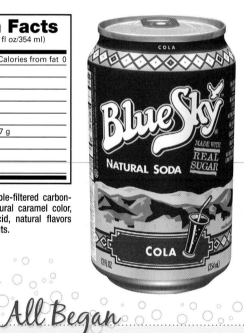

Savvy Pick
Finding a cola that tasted like Coke was like doing our own soda challenge. Every cola has a distinct flavor regardless of your preference. If you are looking for a cleaner option without high-fructose corn syrup, Blue Sky Beverage Cola is a solid competitor that will satisfy your cola craving.

Honorable Mentions

✤ Hansen's Natural
  Cane Soda

✤ Boylan Bottleworks
  Cane Cola

How It All Began

Coca-Cola's formula was invented by a pharmacist named John Pemberton in 1886. Frank Robinson, John's bookkeeper, came up with the name and the logo. Coca-Cola's total sales in its first year of business came to $50. Over the next three years, John sold the formula to another pharmacist for $2,300. Nowadays, 1.6 billion servings of Coca-Cola Company beverages are consumed every day.

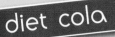
diet cola

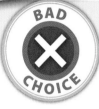
BAD ✗ CHOICE

Diet Pepsi

Aspartame
A 12-ounce can of Diet Pepsi has 177 milligrams of aspartame. In comparison, a packet of Equal contains only 39 milligrams. This just goes to show you how much artificial sweetener actually goes into sweetening a can of diet soda—a lot! That's 4½ packets per can.

Caffeine
Even though caffeine may help you feel more alert in the short-term, in the long-term it will make you feel more tired. Caffeine isn't a stimulant; but rather, it blocks adenosine, a brain chemical that tells you when you are fatigued. It also disrupts the production of melatonin (especially if you drink a caffeinated beverage in the afternoon), the hormone you need to ensure a good night's sleep. Caffeine triggers the fight or flight response, flooding the body with stress hormones including cortisol and adrenaline. Repeatedly triggering the body's stress response causes energy highs and lows, eventually causing "burnout."

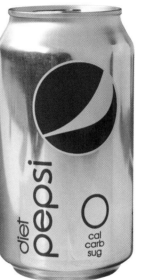

Nutrition Facts
Serving size 1 can (12 fl oz/354 ml)

Calories 0	Calories from fat 0

Total fat 0 g	
Saturated fat 0 g	
Trans fat 0 g	
Cholesterol 0 mg	
Sodium 35 mg	
Total carbohydrates 0 g	
Dietary fiber 0 g	
Sugars 0 g	
Protein 0 g	

INGREDIENTS: carbonated water, caramel color, aspartame, phosphoric acid, potassium benzoate (preservative), caffeine, citric acid, natural flavors. Phenylketonurics: contains phenylalanine.

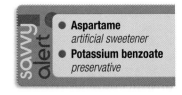

savvy alert

- **Aspartame**
  artificial sweetener
- **Potassium benzoate**
  preservative

tooth truth Sipping sodas throughout the day can result in cavities. The sugar and acids can weaken and permanently damage tooth enamel.

Blue Sky Free Cola

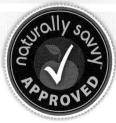

Nutrition Facts
Serving size 1 can (12 fl oz/354 ml)

Calories 0	Calories from fat 0
Total fat 0 g	
Saturated fat 0 g	
Trans fat 0 g	
Cholesterol 0 mg	
Sodium 10 mg	
Total carbohydrates 0 g	
Dietary fiber 0 g	
Sugars 0 g	
Protein 0 g	

INGREDIENTS: triple-filtered carbonated water, erythritol, natural flavors (African Ivory Coast kola nut, South American kola nut oil), caramel color, tartaric acid, Rebiana (stevia extract).

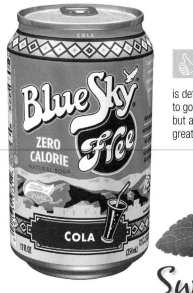

Savvy Pick
If you don't mind drinking a can of chemicals, Diet Pepsi is definitely the way to go. If you prefer to go with something just as refreshing but aspartame free, Blue Sky Free is a great alternative.

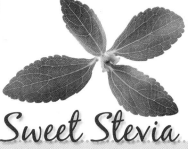

Sweet Stevia

The sweeteners Truvia (developed by Coca-Cola and Cargill) and PureVia (developed by PepsiCo and Whole Earth Sweetener Company) have already replaced aspartame and other dangerous artificial sweeteners in many products, including sodas. They are made from rebaudioside A, an extract from the stevia leaf, as well as erythritol and natural flavors. While Truvia and PureVia may be new to the marketplace, stevia, the plant from which they are derived, has been used as a natural sweetener for thousands of years. Ironically, the FDA does not approve stevia as a food additive (only the extract rebaudioside A).

citrus soda

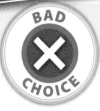

Sprite
Lemon-Lime Soda

Sodium and potassium benzoate

Sodium benzoate and potassium benzoate, both salts of benzoic acid, are preservatives often added to food and drinks. They are the same as far as their functionality—and their dangers to health. There is evidence that sodium and potassium benzoate form benzene, a carcinogen when combined with other acids—including citric acid—which is found in Sprite.

High-fructose corn syrup

In some countries, Sprite is made with real sugar rather than high-fructose corn syrup. While it's more expensive to buy, consumers claim that it tastes much better.

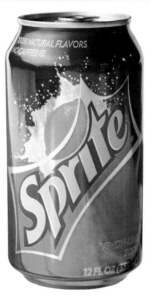

Nutrition Facts
Serving size 1 can (12 fl oz/354 ml)

Calories 140	Calories from fat 0
Total fat 0 g	
Saturated fat 0 g	
Trans fat 0 g	
Cholesterol 0 mg	
Sodium 45 mg	
Total carbohydrates 27 g	
Dietary fiber 0 g	
Sugars 27 g	
Protein 0 g	

INGREDIENTS: carbonated water, high-fructose corn syrup, citric acid, natural flavors, sodium citrate, sodium benzoate (preservative).

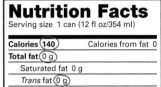

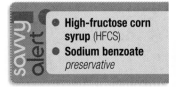

savvy alert
- **High-fructose corn syrup** (HFCS)
- **Sodium benzoate** *preservative*

portion control

Since a can of soda contains 8 teaspoons of sugar, reduce your sugar intake by mixing carbonated water with 100 percent fruit juice. Some combinations to try are cranberry, orange, grape, and peach.

Santa Cruz Organic
Lemon Lime Sparkling Beverage

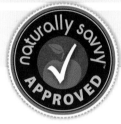

Nutrition Facts
Serving size 1 can (10.5 fl oz/311 ml)

Calories 130	Calories from fat 0
Total fat 0 g	
Saturated fat 0 g	
Trans fat 0 g	
Cholesterol 0 mg	
Sodium 0 mg	
Total carbohydrates 32 g	
Dietary fiber 0 g	
Sugars 32 g	
Protein 0 g	

INGREDIENTS: sparkling filtered water, organic evaporated cane juice, organic lemon and organic lime juice concentrates, organic lemon and organic lime juices, organic natural flavors.

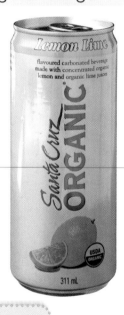

Savvy Pick
Aside from "natural flavors," Sprite's list of synthetic ingredients can't compete with the goodness of Santa Cruz's organic juices and ingredients. In our Savvy opinion, if you're going to ingest 130-odd calories of (let's face it) sugar, you may as well get some nutritional value out of it such as potassium and vitamin C, which comes from the lemon and lime juices. For true lemon-lime refreshment, Santa Cruz is our choice.

Honorable Mentions

❖ Oogavé
Agave Mandarin Key Lime

❖ Izze Esque
Sparkling Limon Juice

WARNING: Bisphenol A

Bisphenol A (BPA) is a chemical used to make the plastic polycarbonate, used in plastic water bottles and to line aluminum cans. This synthetic compound can trick cells into thinking it is the hormone estrogen, which can potentially lead to hormone imbalance and weight gain. It's especially dangerous for babies and pregnant women. Some companies have already taken measures to remove BPA from their packaging, namely baby product manufacturers and Eden Foods' canned tomato products.

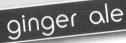

ginger ale

BAD ✕ **CHOICE**

Canada Dry
Ginger Ale

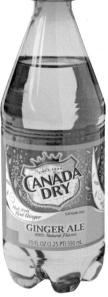

Where's the ginger?
Canada Dry's website (www.canadadry .com) states that its ginger ale is *"made from real ginger,"* but we don't see ginger listed anywhere in the ingredients list. That's because it's lumped under "natural flavors," and the company doesn't divulge how much ginger is actually used. Keep in mind that under FDA guidelines, "natural flavors" does not specify that significant amounts of any ingredient need to be used. We would file this one under "misleading marketing."

Caramel
Caramel is added to soda to give it a rich golden-brown color. The type of caramel used in soda, Caramel IV, is the most worrisome since it's made by reacting sugars with ammonium and sulphite compounds, resulting in the formation of carcinogenic by-products. If soda manufacturers don't switch to safer forms of caramel, we may soon see warning labels on soda cans and bottles.

Nutrition Facts
Serving size 8 fl oz (240 ml)

Calories 90	Calories from fat 0

Total fat 0 g	
Saturated fat 0 g	
Trans fat 0 g	
Cholesterol 0 mg	
Sodium 35 mg	
Total carbohydrates 25 g	
Dietary fiber 0 g	
Sugars 24 g	
Protein 0 g	

INGREDIENTS: carbonated water, high-fructose corn syrup, citric acid, sodium benzoate (preservative), natural flavors, caramel (color).

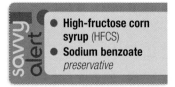

savvy alert
- **High-fructose corn syrup** (HFCS)
- **Sodium benzoate** *preservative*

savvy tip

Well known for soothing nausea, morning sickness, and motion sickness, ginger has also been known to alleviate the sore throat and sinus congestion that often accompany the common cold. The "root" of the ginger plant (which is actually a rhizome, or stem, and not a root) is most useful as a medicine and flavoring.

Hansen's Natural Cane Soda
Ginger Ale

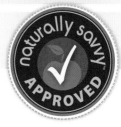

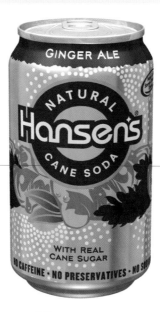

Nutrition Facts
Serving size 1 can (12 fl oz/354 ml)

Calories 170	Calories from fat 0
Total fat 0 g	
Saturated fat 0 g	
Trans fat 0 g	
Cholesterol 0 mg	
Sodium 0 mg	
Total carbohydrates 44 g	
Dietary fiber 0 g	
Sugars 44 g	
Protein 0 g	

INGREDIENTS: pure triple-filtered carbonated water, sugar, citric acid, natural flavors with extracts of Madagascan, Indonesian, or Indian vanilla, natural citrus flavors, extracts of ginger, caramel (color).

Savvy Pick
We love Hansen's exotic-sounding Madagascan vanilla and extracts of ginger (that's real ginger) cane soda—it doesn't contain any HFCS or sodium benzoate—a BIG thumbs-up for us. Hansen's Ginger Ale is higher in calories than Canada Dry, even when you balance out the serving size, but once again it's the ingredients that won us over (not to mention the great taste).

Honorable Mentions

❖ Natural Brew *Reed's Ginger Brew*
❖ GuS Grown-Up Soda
❖ Fresh Ginger *Gingerale by Bruce Cost*

Ginger

The next time you're feeling under the weather, brew a cup of organic ginger tea, add 2 teaspoons of honey, and sip slowly. Try Traditional Medicinals high-quality medicinal grade organic ginger tea for maximum benefits.

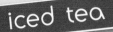

iced tea

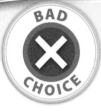

Lipton
Brisk Iced Tea with Lemon

Serving size
Note that one serving size is 8 fluid ounces—which is lower than the amount in an entire bottle.

Phosphoric acid
Phosphoric acid is added to soda to give it a tangy flavor. Excessive intake of phosphorus may interfere with calcium absorption in the body. The average American drinks 46 gallons of soda a year, which makes soft drinks a major source of phosphorus in our diet—and a significant contributor to bone loss.

Sodium polyphosphate
This additive falls under the category of phosphates and is used to regulate acidity in foods and drinks. There are no known negative health effects as a result of ingesting it and it is considered safe.

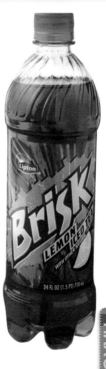

Nutrition Facts
Serving size 8 fl oz (240 ml)

Calories 80	Calories from fat 0
Total fat 0 g	
Saturated fat 0 g	
Trans fat 0 g	
Cholesterol 0 mg	
Sodium 65 mg	
Total carbohydrates 22 g	
Dietary fiber 0 g	
Sugars 22 g	
Protein 0 g	
Caffeine 7 mg	

INGREDIENTS: water, high-fructose corn syrup, citric acid, instant tea, sodium hexametaphosphate and sodium poly-phosphate (to protect flavor), natural flavors, phosphoric acid, sodium benzoate and potassium sorbate (preserve freshness), calcium disodium EDTA (preservative), caramel and Red 40 (color).

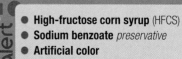

savvy alert
- **High-fructose corn syrup** (HFCS)
- **Sodium benzoate** *preservative*
- **Artificial color**

savvy fact L-theanine, a unique amino acid found in tea, can help you relax without causing drowsiness. In a study of university students, 50 milligrams of L-theanine eased anxiety and increased alpha brain wave activity (the type associated with relaxation) after only forty-five minutes.

Snapple
Lemon Tea

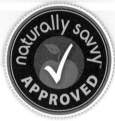

Nutrition Facts
Serving size 8 fl oz (240 ml)

Calories 80	Calories from fat 0
Total fat 0 g	
Saturated fat 0 g	
Trans fat 0 g	
Cholesterol 0 mg	
Sodium 5 mg	
Total carbohydrates 21 g	
Dietary fiber 0 g	
Sugars 21 g	
Protein 0 g	

INGREDIENTS: filtered water, sugar, citric acid, tea, natural flavors.

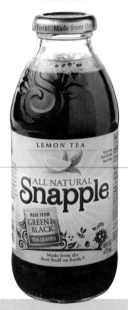

Savvy Pick
By now you know how much we love products with short ingredients lists. Snapple's five easy-to-pronounce ingredients trump Lipton Brisk's long list, which includes HFCS, sodium benzoate, and Red 40.

Green Tea
BENEFITS

Research suggests that many health benefits attributed to tea are largely due to its polyphenols (naturally occurring antioxidants), including epigallocatechin-3-gallate (EGCG), which is the main biologically active component of green tea. One of its proven benefits is its regulatory effect on fat metabolism (weight loss). As little as one cup of green tea—which supplies 50 to 100 mg of ECGC—will provide you with some nutritional benefits. Look for a high-quality brand of tea like Bigelow Tea, Stash Tea, or Choice Organic Tea. If you prefer to take ECGC in supplement form, try abs+ by Genuine Health.

lemonade

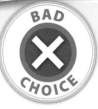

Minute Maid
Lemonade

High-fructose corn syrup
Americans consume approximately 47 teaspoons of caloric sweeteners per day (including HFCS). That's 35 teaspoons more than the daily maximum recommended by the USDA for someone eating a 2,200-calorie diet.

Glycerol of ester gum rosin
Also known as ester gum, this safe food additive is used as an emulsifier to keep oils in suspension in water. It comes from pine trees and is used in all sorts of things: oil paint, paper, soap, printing ink—and food.

Preservatives
Preservatives are added to slow the growth of mold, yeasts, and bacteria so that they can sit on store shelves for months at a time. Potassium sorbate's side effects are minimal; sodium benzoate, however, has been proven to damage DNA.

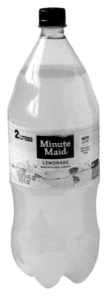

Nutrition Facts
Serving size 8 fl oz (240 ml)

Calories 100	Calories from fat 0

Total fat 0 g	
Saturated fat 0 g	
Trans fat 0 g	
Cholesterol 0 mg	
Sodium 15 mg	
Total carbohydrates 28 g	
Dietary fiber 0 g	
Sugars 28 g	
Protein 0 g	

INGREDIENTS: pure filtered water, high-fructose corn syrup, lemon juice from concentrate. Less than 0.5 percent each of natural flavors, citric acid (provides tartness), modified cornstarch, glycerol of ester gum rosin, sodium benzoate and potassium sorbate and calcium disodium EDTA (to protect taste), Yellow 5 (color).

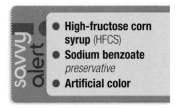

savvy alert

- **High-fructose corn syrup** (HFCS)
- **Sodium benzoate** *preservative*
- **Artificial color**

savvy tip Begin each day by drinking a glass of room-temperature water with a generous squeeze of fresh lemon about 20 minutes before eating or drinking anything else. It will stimulate your energy level *almost* as well as a cup of coffee.

Simply Lemonade

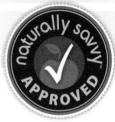

Nutrition Facts

Serving size 8 fl oz (240 ml)

Calories 120	Calories from fat 0
Total fat 0 g	
Saturated fat 0 g	
Trans fat 0 g	
Cholesterol 0 mg	
Sodium 15 mg	
Total carbohydrates 30 g	
Dietary fiber 0 g	
Sugars 28 g	
Protein 0 g	

INGREDIENTS: pure filtered water, natural sugar, lemon juice, natural flavors.

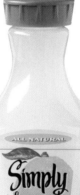

 Savvy Pick
Simply Lemonade is made with the same simple ingredients that you would use to make homemade lemonade. Minute Maid Lemonade's ingredient list reads like a science experiment. Even with 20 extra calories per 8-ounce serving, Simply Lemonade is our preference.

Hello, Yellow

Yellow fruits and vegetables, including lemons, yellow apples, pineapples, yellow watermelon, yellow peppers, and yellow raisins, contain varying amounts of powerful antioxidants such as vitamin C. Include yellow fruits in your diet every day. Even better, mix in some orange, purple, red, and green foods to provide your body with the nutrients it needs.

orange drink

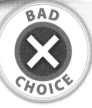

BAD
CHOICE

SunnyD
Tangy Original Citrus Punch

SunnyD downer

The makers of SunnyD created it because their kids didn't like the taste of real orange juice, so they came up with a product in which real fruit juice comprises only 2 percent or less of the ingredients. SunnyD's website states that the artificial sweeteners they use are approved by the FDA. The FDA also approves the artificial colors listed in their ingredients. Just because they're approved doesn't mean they're good for you.

Neotame

The sweetest sweetener ever made, Neotame, is a chemical sweetener that is very similar to aspartame in its composition. Because it is fairly new to the marketplace, more research is needed to determine its safety—but if its effects are anything like those of aspartame, we recommend staying away from it.

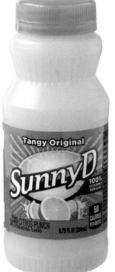

Nutrition Facts
Serving size 8 fl oz (240 ml)

Calories 60	Calories from fat 0
Total fat 0 g	
Saturated fat 0 g	
Trans fat 0 g	
Cholesterol 0 mg	
Sodium 170 mg	
Total carbohydrates 16 g	
Dietary fiber 0 g	
Sugars 14 g	
Protein 0 g	

INGREDIENTS: water, high-fructose corn syrup. Contains 2 percent or less of each: concentrated juices (orange, tangerine, apple, lime, grapefruit), citric acid, ascorbic acid (Vitamin C), thiamine hydrochloride (Vitamin B₁), natural flavors, modified cornstarch, canola oil, sodium citrate, cellulose gum, acesulfame potassium, Neotame, sodium hexametaphosphate, potassium sorbate and sodium benzoate to protect flavor, Yellow 5 and Yellow 6 (color).

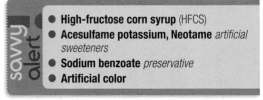

savvy alert
- **High-fructose corn syrup** (HFCS)
- **Acesulfame potassium, Neotame** *artificial sweeteners*
- **Sodium benzoate** *preservative*
- **Artificial color**

savvy tip
If you love orange juice, choose freshly squeezed for the maximum supply of nutrients and antioxidants. And watch your serving size: limit your drink to a half cup or water it down to soften (or buffer) the blood sugar spike.

Capri Sun
Sunrise Orange Wake Up

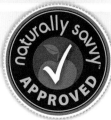

Nutrition Facts
Serving size 6 fl oz (177 ml)

Calories 60	Calories from fat 0
Total fat 0 g	
Saturated fat 0 g	
Trans fat 0 g	
Cholesterol 0 mg	
Sodium 15 mg	
Total carbohydrates 15 g	
Dietary fiber 0 g	
Sugars 15 g	
Protein 0 g	

INGREDIENTS: water, sugar, apple and orange juice concentrates, calcium lactate, citric acid, water-extracted orange juice concentrate, ascorbic acid (vitamin C), natural flavor.

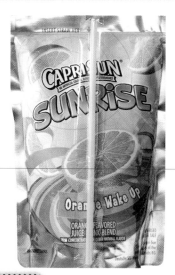

 Savvy Pick
If you aren't a fan of freshly squeezed OJ or don't have time to make it, Capri Sun Sunrise offers a cleaner version of SunnyD. However, we still prefer the real thing. Note: not all the Capri Sun flavors are as clean as Sunrise so read the label carefully when buying other Capri Sun products.

Honorable Mention

✦ R. W. Knudsen Family
Simply Nutritious Morning Blend

Sunny D Vitamin
The Real

The sun helps the body produce vitamin D, and research is exploring this vitamin's positive impact on diseases such as cancer, depression, Parkinson's disease, and obesity. Since natural sunshine comes with risks—namely, skin cancer—if you'd prefer to take a supplement, 200 to 600 IU (international units) of vitamin D_3 is the recommended minimum dose. Speak to your doctor about having a blood test to check your levels of 25-hydroxy D. For a comprehensive look at the benefits of vitamin D, read Dr. Zoltan Rona's book, *Vitamin D: The Sunshine Vitamin*, available from Amazon.

single serve drink mix—cherry

Kool-Aid Singles
Powdered Soft Drink Mix—Cherry

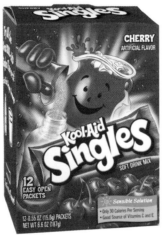

Nutrition Facts
Serving size 8 g (makes 17 fl oz to be added to a water bottle)

Calories 30	Calories from fat 0
Total fat 0 g	
Saturated fat 0 g	
Trans fat 0 g	
Cholesterol 0 mg	
Sodium 0 mg	
Total carbohydrates 7 g	
Dietary fiber 0 g	
Sugars 7 g	
Protein 0 g	

Red 40
This petroleum-based artificial dye has been linked to hyperactivity in children. An adult body might be able to handle more artificial colors, but Kool-Aid products are unmistakably marketed to kids—and that's just not cool.

Sucralose
Splenda is the brand name for the ingredient sucralose. According to the Splenda website (www.splenda.com), *"Splenda is made through a multistep process that starts with sugar and ends as a calorie-free sweetener that the body does not recognize as a carbohydrate and doesn't metabolize."* Nonetheless, an animal study on sucralose showed that this sugar substitute might actually cause weight gain rather than contribute to weight management.

Bottom line
Listen to your body to observe how it reacts when ingesting artificial sweeteners and colors in products such as this one.

INGREDIENTS: sugar, fructose, citric acid (provides tartness). Contains less than 2 percent of each: natural and artificial flavors, ascorbic acid (Vitamin C), Vitamin E acetate, calcium phosphate (prevents caking), acesulfame potassium and sucralose (sweeteners), artificial color, Red 40.

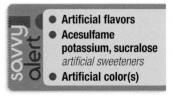

savvy alert
- **Artificial flavors**
- **Acesulfame potassium, sucralose** *artificial sweeteners*
- **Artificial color(s)**

D-I-Y Smoothie Station

Mixed berry smoothie: ½ cup berries, 1 banana, coconut milk, ice. Throw in some ground flaxseeds and fish oil (Nordic Naturals, Barlean's, Carlson, or Ascenta) for a nutrient-rich drink.

Flavrz
Liquid Drink Mix—Cherry Berry

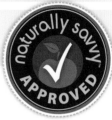

Nutrition Fact
Serving size ½ oz (add to 6–10 oz of water)

Calories 35	Calories from fat 0
Total fat 0 g	
Saturated fat 0 g	
Trans fat 0 g	
Cholesterol 0 mg	
Sodium 0 mg	
Total carbohydrates 8 g	
Dietary fiber 0 g	
Sugars 4 g	
Protein 0 g	

INGREDIENTS: organic apple juice from concentrate (water and organic apple juice concentrate), organic agave syrup, organic evaporated cane juice, water, organic fruit flavors, citric acid, ascorbic acid (Vitamin C), purple carrot extract for color.

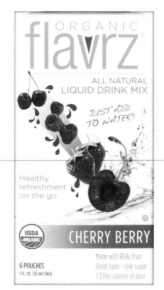

ORGANIC
flavrz
ALL NATURAL
LIQUID DRINK MIX

JUST ADD TO WATER!

Healthy refreshment on the go

USDA ORGANIC

CHERRY BERRY

6 POUCHES
1 FL. OZ. (32 ml) EACH

Made with REAL fruit
Great taste – low sugar
1/3 the calories of juice

Savvy Pick
If you thought Kool-Aid used "real juice" in its ingredients, think again. You have to look pretty hard to find a natural ingredient. Flavrz is made with organic ingredients and uses no artificial sweeteners, yet it has the same number of calories. Your kids will love it.

Açai Berries

Pronounced *a-sigh-ee*, this Brazilian purplish-black berry is widely used in energy-boosting juices, energy bars, and even ice cream. With more antioxidants than cranberry or orange juice, açai is recognized as a top superfood by health experts. Its antioxidants appear to be antibacterial and anti-inflammatory, and they support the cardiovascular system. If that weren't enough, açai berries are also rich in iron and fiber. Enjoy a glass of açai juice and also try antioxidant-rich pomegranate and mangosteen juices.

low-calorie drinks

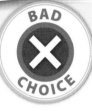

Crystal Light
Pink Lemonade

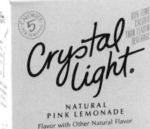
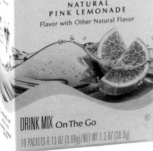

NATURAL
PINK LEMONADE
Flavor with Other Natural Flavor

DRINK MIX On The Go
10 PACKETS-0.13 OZ (3.08g)/NET WT 1.3 OZ (36.8g)

Artificial sweeteners

Why is there so much controversy over artificial sweeteners? Part of the reason is that people react differently to them. While some can handle larger doses without any noticeable reaction, others experience symptoms such as headaches from chewing a piece of gum.

Artificially sweetened drinks

A study of almost 60,000 women found that daily consumption of artificially sweetened drinks appears to increase the risk of delivering babies preterm. Most pregnant women know better than to drink alcohol, but many don't think twice before drinking diet drinks.

Nutrition Facts
Serving size ½ packet

Calories 5	Calories from fat 0

Total fat 0 g	
Saturated fat 0 g	
Trans fat 0 g	
Cholesterol 0 mg	
Sodium 0 mg	
Total carbohydrates 0 g	
Dietary fiber 0 g	
Sugars 0 g	
Protein 0 g	

INGREDIENTS: citric acid, potassium citrate, maltodextrin, aspartame (phenylketonurics: contains phenylalanine), magnesium oxide. Contains less than 2 percent of each: natural flavor, acesulfame potassium, soy lecithin, Red 40 (color).

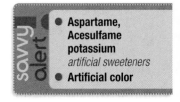

savvy alert
- **Aspartame, Acesulfame potassium**
  artificial sweeteners
- **Artificial color**

savvy tip If you have recurring symptoms that you haven't been able to link to anything in particular, keep a daily food diary to help you identify whether a food or food additive is the cause.

Hansen's Natural Fruit Stix
Lemonade— Strawberry

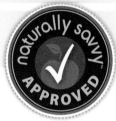

Nutrition Facts

Serving size ½ packet (2 g; makes 8 fl oz/240 ml)

Calories 5	Calories from fat 0 g
Total fat 0 g	
Saturated fat 0 g	
Trans fat 0 g	
Cholesterol 0 mg	
Sodium 20 mg	
Total carbohydrates 1 g	
Dietary fiber 0 g	
Sugars 0 g	
Protein 0 g	

INGREDIENTS: maltodextrin, citric acid, natural flavor, ascorbic acid (vitamin C), stevia extract (rebaudioside A), sodium citrate, vegetable juice powder (color), potassium citrate, carrageenan, calcium phosphate, beta-carotene, calcium silicate, calcium carbonate, sodium bicarbonate.

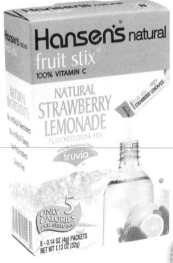

Savvy Pick

Crystal Light might help us drink more water, but to keep the product low-cal, it uses artificial sweeteners. The sweetness of Hansen's comes primarily from the natural sweetener stevia, making it the clear winner.

Honorable Mention

❖ ToGo
Extreme Berries

What is ...?

Stevia

Stevia is a natural, noncaloric sweetener that can be used as a replacement for sugar in food and drinks. Stevia extracts, called steviosides, can be up to three hundred times sweeter than table sugar. Almost one hundred nutrients have been identified in stevia, so it is considered a healthy alternative sweetener. The sweetener can be used for coffee, tea, smoothies, and desserts, and is available in both powder and liquid forms.

vitamin-enriched water

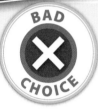

Propel
Blueberry Pomegranate

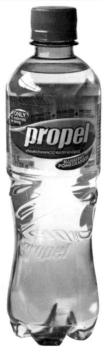

Artificial sweeteners

Water is an essential nutrient, and the idea of enriching water with vitamins is brilliant. Adding dangerous artificial sweeteners and a lot of sugar, however, ruins a good thing, especially when the additive in question is acesulfame potassium, which many health experts feel is one of the riskiest artificial sweeteners.

Is sucralose safe?

This has yet to be established. According to osteopath and author Dr. Joseph Mercola, there have only been six human studies on this artificial sweetener to date, with the longest one lasting for a period of only three months. He believes it is not safe and we concur.

Nutrition Facts
Serving size 8 fl oz (240 ml)

Calories 0	Calories from fat 0
Total fat 0 g	
Saturated fat 0 g	
Trans fat 0 g	
Cholesterol 0 mg	
Sodium 80 mg	
Total carbohydrates 0 g	
Dietary fiber 0 g	
Sugars 0 g	
Protein 0 g	

INGREDIENTS: water, citric acid, sodium hexametaphosphate (to protect flavor), natural flavor, potassium sorbate (preservative), ascorbic acid (Vitamin C), sucralose, sodium citrate, potassium citrate, acesulfame potassium, niacinamide (Vitamin B_5), calcium disodium EDTA (preservative), Vitamin E acetate, calcium pantothenate (Vitamin B_5), pyridoxine hydrochloride (Vitamin B_6).

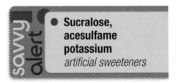

savvy alert
- **Sucralose, acesulfame potassium**
  artificial sweeteners

Glaceau Vitamin Water XXX
Açai-Blueberry-Pomegranate

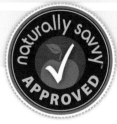

Nutrition Facts

Serving size 8 fl oz (240 ml)

Calories 50	Calories from fat 0
Total fat 0 g	
Saturated fat 0 g	
Trans fat 0 g	
Cholesterol 0 mg	
Sodium 0 mg	
Total carbohydrates 13 g	
Dietary fiber 0 g	
Sugars 13 g	
Protein 0 g	

INGREDIENTS: reverse-osmosis water, crystalline fructose, cane sugar. Less than 0.5 percent of each of: citric acid, ascorbic acid (Vitamin C), fruit and vegetable juice (color), natural flavor, berry and fruit extracts (apple, pomegranate, açai, blueberry), magnesium lactate (electrolyte), niacinamide (Vitamin B_3), calcium pantothenate (Vitamin B_5), calcium lactate (electrolyte), potassium phosphate (electrolyte), beta-carotene, pyridoxine hydrochloride (Vitamin B_6), cyanocobalamin (Vitamin B_{12}), manganese citrate, gum acacia.

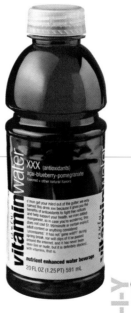

Savvy Pick

Propel may have fewer calories, but artificial sweeteners are a huge Naturally Savvy no-no. Kudos to Vitamin Water for using antioxidant-rich ingredients, solidifying them as our pick.

Honorable Mentions

✢ Ex Drinks
  Aqua Vitamins

✢ Oxylent
  Oxygenating Multivitamin Supplement Drink

D-I-Y Vitamin Water

Make your own vitamin-enriched water. Cut up some fresh-tasting vegetables—such as cucumbers, celery, or red peppers, or lemons, limes, or oranges—in a container and fill it with water. Allow it to sit overnight in the refrigerator. Remove the vegetables and drink the water. If you'd like to sweeten your drink, add some honey.

sports drinks

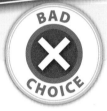

Powerade
Mountain Berry Blast

 High-fructose corn syrup
The battle against HFCS took a huge turn in the right direction when PepsiCo announced that it was removing high-fructose corn syrup from its Gatorade products. Hopefully, Powerade will do the same.

Electrolytes
Electrolytes are minerals that carry electrical impulses from cell to cell. They include sodium, calcium, potassium, chlorine, phosphate and magnesium. When you exercise heavily, you lose electrolytes in your sweat (particularly sodium and potassium). Replacing electrolytes is essential for keeping up the electrolyte concentration of your body fluids, especially if you're active—which is why many sports drinks add them.

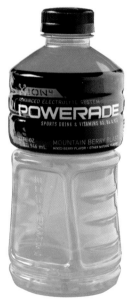

Nutrition Facts
Serving size 8 fl oz (240 ml)

Calories 50	Calories from fat 0
Total fat 0 g	
Saturated fat 0 g	
Trans fat 0 g	
Cholesterol 0 mg	
Sodium 100 mg	
Total carbohydrates 14 g	
Dietary fiber 0 g	
Sugars 14 g	
Protein 0 g	

INGREDIENTS: water, high-fructose corn syrup, citric acid, sodium chloride (electrolyte), natural flavors, potassium citrate (electrolyte), modified food starch, magnesium chloride (electrolyte), calcium chloride (electrolyte), potassium phosphate (electrolyte), calcium disodium EDTA (preservative), coconut oil, niacinamide (vitamin B_3), Blue 1 (color), pyridoxine hydrochloride (vitamin B_6), cyanocobalamin (vitamin B_{12}).

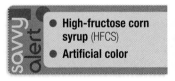

savvy alert
- **High-fructose corn syrup** (HFCS)
- **Artificial color**

sports drinks

Don't wait until the day of the marathon to try a new sports drink or energy bar! Different bodies respond differently to foods and beverages, so experiment with energy boosters or carb boosters during your training—well in advance of game day—to determine how your body will react to a new substance.

R. W. Knudsen Family
Mixed Berry Recharge

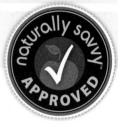

Nutrition Facts

Serving size 8 fl oz (240 ml)

Calories 70	Calories from fat 0
Total fat 0 g	
Saturated fat 0 g	
Trans fat 0 g	
Cholesterol 0 mg	
Sodium 25 mg	
Total carbohydrates 18 g	
Dietary fiber 0 g	
Sugars 17 g	
Protein 0 g	

INGREDIENTS: filtered water, white grape, apple raspberry, strawberry, and pineapple juice concentrates, natural flavor, fruit and vegetable juices (color), sea salt.

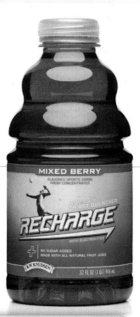

Savvy Pick

Considering all the technology that goes into developing a sports drink, Knudsen managed to create one using very simple ingredients. The natural minerals in sea salt supply a wider array of electrolytes, while providing less sodium than Powerade, and it's naturally colored with juices. For all of the above, Knudsen gets our Savvy Seal of Approval™.

Honorable Mentions

❖ LIV
Organic Sport Drink

❖ Clif
Quench Sport Drink

❖ Oxylent
Oxygenating Multivitamin Supplement Drink

Coconut Water

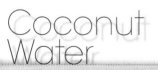

With more electrolytes than leading sports drinks and fifteen times the potassium (almost as much as in two small bananas) coconut water, the clear fluid from green coconuts, keeps your body hydrated and prevents cramping. Staying hydrated helps you to stay alert and energized. Some of our favorite brands are Vita Coco, Zico, and O.N.E.

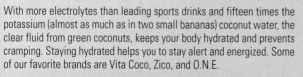
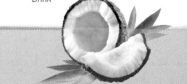

Acesulfame potassium: Also known as acesulfame K or ace K and marketed as Sweet One and Sunett, ace K is a calorie-free artificial sweetener found in over five thousand products worldwide. It is used in chewing gum, diet sodas, and light fruit drinks, and because it is heat stable, acesulfame potassium is used as a replacement for sugar in desserts and baked goods. As a sweetener, it is 200 times sweeter than table sugar (sucrose). Even though ace K was approved by the FDA for consumption in 1988, this sweetener has not been properly tested to determine its safety for human consumption. To date, the FDA has not required further testing, even though early studies indicated that the additive may cause cancer in animals. Acesulfame potassium is not metabolized or stored in the body.

Acids: Food acids are added to enhance flavors and also act as preservatives and antioxidants. Common food acids include vinegar, citric acid (from citrus fruits), tartaric acid (from grapes), fumaric acid, and malic acid (from apples). These natural acids are considered safe for human consumption.

> **Adipic acid:** The food industry uses adipic acid, a precursor to the production of nylon, as an acidulant in gelatins, bottled beverages, gelatin desserts, and powdered fruit concentrates. It gives food a tart flavor, and its low pH prevents the growth of some microorganisms that cause food decay.

> **Citric acid:** Most abundantly present in citrus fruits such as lemons, oranges, and grapefruits. It is not the same as vitamin C (ascorbic acid). In food manufacturing, it can be produced from many different plant sources, including corn. Citric acid brings out the flavor of other ingredients and imparts a tangy or tart flavor to beverages. It is also used to adjust the acidity of beverages to improve their flavor and extend their shelf life.

> **Malic acid:** A fruit acid extracted from apples and widely used in the food industry to add a tart and sour flavor to food. Malic acid is essential in the formation of ATP, one of the body's energy sources. Research suggests promising health benefits from this substance; for instance, malic acid, in combination with magnesium, may be helpful for those with fibromyalgia.

Annatto color (natural color annatto E160b): Annatto is a natural yellow-red plant extract used to dye foods, textiles, and body care products. Its primary use is as a red food coloring in a wide assortment of foods, including cereals, preserved meats, cheeses, and sweets. Annatto is the only natural color known to cause as many adverse effects as artificial colors. Children seem to be especially sensitive to annatto. Adverse reactions can include skin, gastrointestinal, respiratory, and central nervous system effects. On labels, it may appear as annatto, annatto color, or annatto extract.

Antioxidants (food grade): Antioxidants are added to food to slow the oxidation of fats and oils, colorings, and flavorings. Oxidation leads to rancidity (spoilage), flavor changes, and loss of color. Examples of antioxidants include BHA, BHT, and TBHQ. (*See definitions for specific health issues.*)

Artificial butter flavor: This is a mixture containing more than one hundred chemicals, typically including diacetyl and acetoin. Factory workers involved in the production of microwave popcorn have developed bronchiolitis obliterans, a life-threatening inflammatory lung disease, from exposure to diacetyl. The lung disease is also referred to as diacetyl-induced bronchiolitis obliterans (DIBO) or simply Popcorn Worker's Lung. Studies show that diacetyl is toxic to rats, causing lung cell damage upon exposure to the chemical. Diacetyl is also found in ice cream, candy, and baked goods, and it can be hidden in the ingredients list as "artificial flavor." Acetoin is an aroma carrier used in flavor preparations and may also be responsible for Popcorn Worker's Lung. In 2007, manufacturers began switching to less toxic ingredients for use in artificial butter flavor.

Artificial color: Artificial food dyes contain various chemicals and are commonly derived from petroleum products. All food and drink labels must list the artificial colors they contain. To denote food coloring agents, colors are assigned FD&C (Federal Food, Drug and Cosmetic) numbers, which are regulated by the Food and Drug Administration. In the United States, the FDA approves the following seven artificial colorings for general use in food:

- FD&C Blue No. 1—Brilliant Blue FCF, E133 (blue shade). Found in beverages, candy, baked goods. Inadequately tested; suggestions of a small cancer risk.

- FD&C Blue No. 2—Indigotine, E132 (dark blue shade). Found in pet food, beverages, candy.

- FD&C Green No. 3—Fast Green FCF, E143 (bluish-green shade). This dye is rarely used.

- FD&C Red No. 3—Erythrosine. High doses have been shown to cause cancer in lab animals.

- FD&C Red No. 40—Allura Red, E129 (red shade). Made mostly from petroleum, this dye can cause allergy-like reactions and has been linked to hyperactivity in children. Also a potential carcinogen.

- FD&C Yellow No. 5—Tartrazine, E102 (yellow shade). Found in soft drinks, energy drinks, cotton candy, flavored chips, cereals, cake mixes, pastries, sports drinks, and other convenience foods. Reactions may include rash, skin allergies, asthma, or runny nose. Linked to hyperactivity in children.

- FD&C Yellow No. 6—Sunset Yellow, E110 (orange shade). Also known as Sunset Yellow FCF. Found in DayQuil capsules, Extra Strength Tylenol, fortune cookies, some red sauces, chips, and yellow, orange, and red food products. Linked to allergies, nausea, nasal congestion, and hyperactivity in children.

The above are known as primary colors. When they are mixed to produce other colors, those colors are known as secondary colors.

Artificial flavor: Additives designed to mimic the taste of natural ingredients. Artificial flavors are a cheap way for manufacturers to make something taste like strawberry, for example, without actually using strawberries. They are typically found in processed, refined foods and are known to cause allergic and behavioral reactions. Unfortunately, the FDA does not require flavor companies to disclose ingredients as long as all the ingredients have been deemed "Generally Recognized as Safe." This protects the proprietary formulas of the companies that produce artificial flavors, but it allows for many chemicals to be hidden under the word *flavor* on the ingredients list (for example, "artificial strawberry flavor").

Artificial vanilla flavor: *See* Vanillin.

Aspartame: An artificial sweetener used in many diet foods and soft drinks. It is composed of 50 percent phenylalanine, 40 percent aspartic acid, and 10 percent methanol, a substance that converts to deadly neurotoxins. Reported side effects of aspartame include headaches, dizziness, behavioral changes, convulsions, diarrhea, memory loss, itching, hives, and possible brain damage in infants.

Autolyzed yeast extract: *See* Glutamic acid.

Barley malt: A natural sweetener made from sprouted barley. The dark, sweet, thick liquid is composed mainly of maltose. Sometimes used in malted milks.

Benzoates (sodium, potassium, calcium benzoate): Benzoates are antimicrobial preservatives used in foods and beverages to maintain flavor and prevent spoilage. Benzoates are linked to allergic reactions, and cancer.

Beta-carotene: An antioxidant found in many colorful fruits and vegetables. It is used as a food color for yellow to orange shades. It is a safe food additive.

BHA (butylated hydroxyanisole) and BHT (butylated hydroxytoluene): BHA and BHT are two closely related preservatives that are added to foods containing fats and oils to prevent oxidation, slow rancidity, and prolong shelf life. They are often used together. BHA and BHT are found in many foods, including cereals, instant dehydrated potatoes, frozen dinners, baked goods, chewing gum, beer, and some fruit drinks. BHA and BHT have been known to affect the nervous system and cause behavioral problems in children. BHT may convert hormones and oral contraceptives into carcinogens.

Brown rice syrup: A natural sweetener made from cultured rice (usually naturally fermented), broken down by enzymes, strained and cooked to a syrup-like consistency.

Calcium benzoate: *See* Benzoates.

Calcium caseinate: *See* Casein.

Calcium disodium EDTA: Calcium disodium EDTA, or calcium disodium ethylenediaminetetraacetic acid, is an ingredient that is widely used in the food industry as a preservative and stabilizer. Calcium disodium EDTA helps to prevent oxidation of beverages, stabilize flavor oils, prevent discoloration, and help preserve vitamins and minerals. *See* EDTA *for more information.*

Calcium sorbate: *See* Sorbates.

Calcium stearate: A type of salt, this ingredient is used in food as an anticaking agent, binder, emulsifier, filler, and foaming or whipping agent. While there are no reports of toxicity, it has not been thoroughly tested for use in foods.

Calcium sulfate: A calcium salt abundant in nature. In layman's terms, calcium sulfate is chalk. It's added to processed foods such as tofu as a coagulant to prevent curdling and to commercial baked goods as a filler. It also increases the amount of calcium in a product.

Caramel color: *See* Natural coloring.

Carrageenan: *See* Gums.

Carnauba wax: A vegetable wax that comes from the leaves of the Brazilian carnauba palm tree (*Copernicia cerifera*), carnauba wax is used to coat candy, frosting, and gum. It is also used as a coating for floors and cars. It has been known to cause allergic reactions when used in cosmetics.

Carob: This Mediterranean fruit has a naturally sweet and toasty flavor. It has been used as an alternative to chocolate. Carob is a natural fruit and is caffeine free.

Casein: The principal protein in milk. It is a nutritious protein containing adequate amounts of all the essential amino acids. If you are allergic or intolerant to casein, read food labels carefully. It is used in some "nondairy" and "vegetarian" foods. On food labels, casein can also be listed as caseinate, calcium caseinate, ammonia caseinate, magnesium caseinate, potassium caseinate, and sodium caseinate.

Cellulose: *See* Functional fibers.

Chelating agents: A group of ingredients used in food to trap trace amounts of metal atoms that would otherwise cause food to discolor or go rancid. See *EDTA* for an example of a chelating agent.

Citric acid: *See* Acids.

Cocoa, alkalized cocoa: Cocoa is available two ways: natural and alkalized, the second of which is also known as dutched or dutch process. Natural cocoa has nothing added to it and retains its rich, slightly bitter taste. Alkalized or dutched cocoa uses hydroxide to neutralize the acids in the cocoa, producing a less bitter and smoother taste but causing cocoa to lose up to 90 percent of its antioxidants.

Cocoa butter: Cocoa butter is the natural, cream-colored vegetable fat extracted from cocoa beans during the process of making chocolate and cocoa powder. Even though the word *butter* is in its name, it does not contain dairy ingredients of any kind.

Coconut oil: The type used in food manufacturing is called RBD, "refined, bleached and deodorized." The processed oil is sometimes confused with organic virgin cold-pressed coconut oil, a health-promoting oil with a variety of benefits. Organic coconut oil is suitable for cooking and may be purchased at natural product stores and most supermarkets.

Confectioners' glaze, pure food glaze (shellac): A clear coating used to protect the quality of candy. Confectioners' glaze is made with lac, the resin (waste product) produced by the lac beetle that thrives on various host trees and shrubs in India, Myanmar, and Thailand. The lac beetle is not harmed in any way in the harvesting of lac.

Corn syrup: Used as a sweetener to replace sugar in processed foods. Consisting mostly of dextrose, it is a sweet, thick liquid made by treating cornstarch with acids or enzymes. Corn syrup contains no nutritional value other than calories and, like most other forms of sugar, promotes tooth decay.

Date sugar: A natural sweetener made from pulverized, generally unrefined dates, it contains sucrose, glucose, and fructose. It is low in grams of sugar per teaspoon and low in calories.

DATEM (diacetyl tartaric acid ester of monoglyceride): An emulsifier used primarily in baking as a dough modifier, it is also found in margarine, mayonnaise, biscuits, and dressings. This emulsifier can be listed on the ingredients list simply as DATEM. A 2002 study by the Joint FAO/WHO Expert Committee on Food Additives (JECFA) suggested that DATEM at low to moderate doses in rats may cause a stiffening of the heart and enlargement of the adrenal glands. High concentrations of DATEM may decrease the body's ability to use important nutrients such as calcium.

Dextrose: A sugar and corn derivative, dextrose is added to foods as a sweetener. Since glucose and dextrose share the same chemical formula, some companies use the word *dextrose* in place of glucose in their nutritional facts because they believe that consumers view the word *glucose* in a negative light, according to a letter published in the *British Medical Journal*. The average American consumes about 25 pounds of dextrose per year (and a total of about 150 pounds per year of all refined sugars).

Dipotassium phosphate: A food additive added to processed products to control acidity and prevent the food from coagulating, or clumping. You might find it in a snack food that has a cheesy or creamy property.

Disodium guanylate and disodium inosinate: These flavor enhancers work synergistically with monosodium glutamate (MSG) and are hardly ever used in food processing without it.

Disodium phosphate: *See* Phosphoric acid, phosphates.

EDTA (ethylenediaminetetraacetic acid): Added to canned foods to trap metal impurities, maintaining the product's quality. This chelating agent has been found to be toxic to cells and potentially carcinogenic in lab animals. EDTA is also a persistent organic pollutant; it collects in groundwater and has the potential to carry heavy metals back into our drinking water.

Emulsifiers: Molecules that attract both oil and water, emulsifiers enable foods with fat and water components to remain mixed together to make food look more appealing and give the food a consistent texture. Emulsifiers occur in nature (eggs contain a natural emulsifier), but there are also many chemically produced emulsifiers that may affect human health in various ways. The most commonly used emulsifiers are lecithin (E322) and the monoglycerides and diglycerides of fatty acids (E471).

Ester of rosin: This natural substance, collected from longleaf pine trees, is used in citrus-flavored drinks as an emulsifier, allowing the concentrated flavoring oils from lemons, limes, and oranges to mix with other fluids. Although there is no evidence of health risk with use of this natural emulsifier, the safety of glycerol esters of gum rosin—made by esterification of refined gum rosin—as a food additive is currently under review by the European Food Safety Authority (EFSA).

Fractionated palm oil: *See* Palm oil.

Fructose: Fructose is a natural sugar found in fruit. When it appears on a food label, however, it's more likely to be one of the favorite by-products of corn production. Look for these sweeteners that are likely to contain fructose: high-fructose corn syrup, corn syrup, corn syrup solids, corn sweetener, and fruit sweetener. Fructose is sweeter tasting than regular sucrose (table sugar). Consuming too much fructose at once (even from fruit) seems to overwhelm the body's capacity to process it. When glucose enters the bloodstream, the body releases insulin to help regulate it. Fructose, on the other hand, is processed in the liver, where it's either converted to glycogen (the storage form of glucose) or is used to produce triglycerides. The body is more likely to convert fructose to triglycerides in those with a carbohydrate-rich diet, contributing to weight gain. A diet high in fructose may lead to:

- High blood triglycerides, a major risk factor for heart disease.

- Overeating or weight gain. Fructose circumvents the normal appetite signaling system, so appetite-regulating hormones aren't triggered, and you're left feeling unsatisfied.

- Insulin resistance, which can lead to type 2 diabetes.

Functional fibers: While most of us are aware of the nutritional role fiber plays—regulating bowel function, balancing blood sugar, and drawing cholesterol and toxins out of the body—many fibers are used in food manufacturing as additives. Functional fibers are most often used to draw water into a food to improve its texture, to extend a food's shelf life, or to enhance nutritional value. Their versatility allows them to function as thickening agents, stabilizers, binders, gelling agents, and more. Some functional fibers have been heavily processed and should be avoided. These include methylcellulose, hydroxypropyl cellulose, carboxymethylcellulose, and propylene glycol alginate. If you're a label reader, you will likely recognize the following fibers.

> **Alginate:** Derived from algae and seaweed, alginate has chelating properties, latching onto toxins and moving them through the intestinal tract and out of the body. As a food additive, alginates act as stabilizers and impart a creamy texture to processed foods. You'll find alginate in cereal bars, ice cream, salad dressings, cheese spreads, and frozen dinners. Propylene glycol alginate, a chemically modified algin, thickens acidic foods (soda pop, salad dressing) and can stabilize the foam in beer.

> **Cellulose (sodium carboxymethyl cellulose):** The outer layer, or peel of plants. In the food industry, it is used as an anticaking agent, emulsifier, stabilizer, thickener, and gelling agent. It is also used to replace fat in some salad dressings and sauces.

Methylcellulose: Derived from cellulose, methylcellulose is a chemical compound. It is produced by heating cellulose with a harsh solution (for example, sodium hydroxide, the same active ingredient used in Drano) and treating it with methyl chloride. It is used as an emulsifier and thickener in sauces and salad dressings, and as a thickener and stabilizer in ice cream, where it helps prevent ice crystals from forming. It is also sold as an over-the-counter laxative to help relieve constipation. Methylcellulose should be avoided.

Gelatin: A thickening and gelling agent, gelatin is a protein obtained from the connective tissue of animals and fish. Aside from protein, it has little nutritional value. Although allergy to gelatin is rare, reactions may include hives, low blood pressure, runny nose, dizziness, and anaphylaxis.

Glucono delta-lactone: Used to regulate acidity and color in many foods, including baking powder, this safe additive is prepared by fermentation of corn.

Glutamic acid, free glutamic acid: Free glutamic acid is a flavor enhancer that gives food a savory flavor. It is an ingredient in over forty flavor additives, including sodium caseinate, autolyzed yeast, yeast extract, torula yeast, hydrolyzed protein, and monosodium glutamate. Glutamic acid acts as a neurotransmitter and excitotoxin. Because of this, it can cause neurological symptoms in some people, such as headaches.

Glycerol, glycerin: Used in foods and beverages as a filler for low-fat products and as a popular humectant (which means that it helps retain moisture) for baked goods. Glycerol is also used in many personal-care products, including soap and shampoo, so it is a hard ingredient to avoid if you are sensitive to it. Reported allergic reactions include skin irritation, gastrointestinal symptoms, shortness of breath, and even swelling of the tongue or face.

Gums: Most gums derive from various natural sources, including seeds, tree sap, and seaweed. In food manufacturing, they may be added as thickening agents and stabilizers to a wide range of foods; for example, they are used to prevent sugar crystals from forming in candy, form a gel in pudding, and keep oil and water mixed together in salad dressings. According to the Center for Science in the Public Interest, gums are poorly tested but likely safe. Carrageenan, locust bean gum, gum arabic, guar gum, and xanthan gum are among the most widely used in the food industry.

Carrageenan: An extract from seaweed that serves a variety of purposes in processed food. It thickens, emulsifies (*see* Emulsifiers), and gives texture to foods. Since carrageenan is 100 percent animal free, it is used in place of gelatin in vegetarian products. Although it has not been researched heavily, it has been shown to induce ulcerative colitis in lab animals.

Locust bean gum: Obtained from the seeds of carob beans. It is commonly used as a thickener, stabilizer, and gelling agent in cream cheese, ice creams, fruit preparations, and salad dressings.

Gum arabic, gum acacia: A natural food stabilizer. Its low viscosity, high emulsification, and adhesion properties make it an excellent ingredient in bakery products, meal replacers, and coatings of some cereals, snacks, and confections. Gum arabic also has industrial applications and is sometimes used in paints, glues, and textiles.

Guar gum: Used as a thickener, stabilizer, and plasticizer in dairy products, baking, meat items, frozen foods, sauces, salad dressings, and cosmetics.

Tara gum: A natural gum made by grinding the endosperm of the seeds of the tara tree (*Cesalpinia spinosa lin*). The plant is native to South America, where it grows as a tree or bush. It has a gelling effect and increases the gelling properties of agar and carrageenan.

Xanthan gum: Is the result of the fermentation of sugars by the bacteria *Xanthamonas campestris*. Xanthan gum is often added to products that have gelatinous properties. It's also used as a thickener, stabilizer, emulsifier, and binding agent in the preparation of sauces, salad dressings, and dairy products. Xanthan gum is often derived from corn. Individuals with corn allergies are encouraged to contact the manufacturers before consuming xanthan gum in a product.

High-fructose corn syrup (HFCS): An inexpensive sweetener that has largely replaced ordinary sugar in soft drinks and many processed foods. It is highly processed, made by treating corn syrup with chemicals to convert a portion of its glucose molecules into fructose. The result is a product that is sweeter than sugar and much less expensive to produce. HFCS is linked to elevated cholesterol, obesity, and metabolic syndrome. This dangerous sweetener should be avoided.

Hydrogenated starch hydrolysate: A family of products that includes glucose syrups and sugar alcohol syrups. (*See* Sugar alcohols.) They are used as sugar-reduced or sugar-free sweeteners. Often this type of sweetener is derived from corn. While the compounds have been studied in relation to tooth decay, hydrogenated starch hydrolysate has not been widely studied as a food additive.

Hydrolyzed vegetable protein (HVP): Soybean or other vegetable protein that has been chemically broken down to the amino acids of which it is composed. HVP enhances the natural flavor of food and is used in soups, broths, sauces, and spice blends. It is a source of glutamate. Also known as hydrolyzed protein, hydrolyzed corn protein, and hydrolyzed milk protein.

Inulin: A soluble fiber extracted from chicory root. One of the most popular recent health trends is to add inulin to packaged foods (pasta, bread, yogurt), beverages, and even pet food! Inulin acts as a probiotic in the intestines, while binding and removing cholesterol, fat, and dangerous hormones along the way. As a fiber supplement, inulin completely dissolves in water and has no flavor.

Lactose: A naturally occurring sugar in the milk of mammals. It is used as a food additive to produce a sweeter, creamier taste. Lactose intolerance, a common food intolerance, occurs due to a lack of enzymes needed to break down this milk sugar. Symptoms may include cramping, bloating, gas, and diarrhea.

Malic acid: *See* Acids.

Maltodextrin: A polysaccharide used as a thickener and stabilizer for foods such as puddings, desserts, cheese products, and ice cream. It can be produced from any kind of starch. In the United States, this starch is usually corn or potato, while in Europe maltodextrin is commonly derived from barley or wheat. The website Celiac.com (www.celiac.com) deems maltodextrin to be a safe gluten-free food. Tapioca maltodextrin is becoming a popular additive because it is tasteless and odorless.

Margarine: *See* Partially hydrogenated oil.

Modified starch: Used in processed foods to improve their consistency and keep solids suspended. Starch and modified starches sometimes replace more nutritious ingredients, such as fruit.

Molasses: A natural sweetener. The dark brown syrup that remains after sugar has been processed. Blackstrap molasses contains iron and traces of vitamins and minerals.

Monosodium glutamate (MSG): Used to enhance flavor in foods, MSG is one of the most complained about additives. A reaction to MSG is actually a reaction to free glutamic acid, which is also found in these additives: isolated protein source, autolyzed yeast, hydrolyzed vegetable protein, hydrolyzed yeast, vegetable powder, natural flavors, glutamate, caseinate, texturized vegetable protein (TVP), and yeast extract. MSG is best known as an additive in Chinese food, but it is also used in garlic and onion powder, bouillon, soup stock, seasoning for potato chips and popcorn, and breaded foods such as chicken nuggets. Common symptoms related to ingestion of MSG include headache, asthma, chest pains, diarrhea, blurred vision, fatigue, hot flashes, numbness around the face, sweating, palpitations, and urinary discomfort.

Natural coloring: Natural food color is any dye derived from a natural source, including a vegetable, animal, or mineral. Natural dyes can color food, drugs, cosmetics, or any part of the human body. The following are examples of natural food colors:

- Natural types of caramel color made from caramelized sugar.

- Annatto (E160b), a yellow-red dye made from the seed of the achiote. (See *Annatto color* for more information.)

- Carmine, a red dye derived from the cochineal insect *Dactylopius coccus*. This is listed as carmine on food labels—*but you're still eating bugs*. More important, while it's safe for most people, carmine has been known to cause severe, even life-threatening allergic reactions in rare cases.

- Betanin, which is extracted from beets.

- Turmeric, saffron, paprika, elderberry juice, black carrot juice.

Nitrates and nitrites: Nitrites slow spoilage and give a pink color to pork and cured meats such as sausage, hot dogs, bacon, ham, and lunch meats. These chemicals combine with stomach fluids to form nitrosamines, which are carcinogenic. Some companies now add ascorbic acid (vitamin C) or erythorbic acid to bacon to inhibit nitrosamine formation. Choose fresh meat over luncheon meat and look for organic or natural meats that are free of nitrates and nitrites. When processed meat with carcinogenic preservatives are consumed, combine with a food rich in vitamin C to help reduce the formation of nitrosamines.

Olestra: An additive used to make low-fat or fat-free foods, olestra (brand name, Olean) can cause diarrhea, abdominal cramps, gas, and other adverse effects. It can also interfere with the absorption of health-protective fat-soluble vitamins and antioxidants.

Oligofructose: Produced from chicory root, oligofructose is slightly sweet and provides less than half as many calories per gram as fructose or other sugar. It also promotes the growth of beneficial bifidus bacteria.

Palm oil: Palm oil is used to replace partially hydrogenated oil (trans fat) in many foods. Palm trees produce a fleshy fruit from which two oils are extracted: palm oil from the fruit (also called palm fruit oil) and palm kernel oil from the pit. Of the two, palm fruit oil is healthier, with less saturated fat and more antioxidants (in particular, vitamin E). Palm kernel oil is extremely high in saturated fat (about 80 percent). Fractionated palm oil—the worst form of palm oil—and modified palm oil are further processed, are highest in saturated fats, and are not much better than the partially hydrogenated oil they are intended to replace.

Partially hydrogenated oil: Added to foods to make them more stable and increase shelf life. In production, liquid vegetable oil is exposed to hydrogen gas at high heat and high pressure in the presence of a metal catalyst to make the oil more stable and solid. A by-product of hydrogenation is trans fat, which promotes heart disease by increasing the amount of "bad" (LDL) cholesterol in the blood and decreasing the "good" (HDL) cholesterol. This is one of the most dangerous food additives. The FDA has enforced the labeling of trans fat since January 2006.

Pectin: A highly soluble fiber found under the peel of many fruits, vegetables, and legumes. Because of the fiber's ability to hold water, the food industry uses pectin (from citrus peel or apple) as a gelling agent to make jam and as a thickener. Look for it on labels of many foods, including yogurt, many desserts, and even ketchup.

Phosphoric acid, phosphates: An acidulant that adds a pleasant tartness to certain beverages and acts as a preservative, it is often added to soft drinks. Phosphoric acid contains phosphorus, an essential nutrient and one of the basic elements of nature. Too many sources of phosphate from one's diet, however, can interfere with calcium absorption. Here are some other types of phosphates:

- *Sodium phosphate* is a generic term that may refer to any sodium salt of phosphoric acid, such as disodium phosphate, a white powder used as an anticaking additive, texturizer, and stabilizer in powdered products. Sodium phosphates are commonly added to food and may serve a variety of purposes. They have been well studied and are generally considered safe when used as a food additive.

- Sodium aluminum phosphate is a leavening agent.

- Calcium and ammonium phosphates are used in baking as leavening agents.

- Sodium acid pyrophosphate prevents discoloration in potatoes and sugar syrups, and is used as a leavening agent in baked goods.

Polydextrose: Approved for use in food in the United States in 1994, polydextrose is made by combining dextrose (corn sugar) with sorbitol. It can be found in a number of different types of low-calorie sweets such as puddings, frozen desserts, and hard candy. As a thickening agent, polydextrose is used in homemade puddings and dessert sauces. Polydextrose partially ferments in the colon and appears to provide the benefits of dietary fiber without abdominal distention and cramping; however, this ingredient tends to be added to products alongside unhealthy ingredients, and so excessive consumption may cause diarrhea in sensitive individuals.

Polyglycerol polyricinoleate (PGPR): An emulsifier and low-cost replacement for cocoa butter in chocolate bars. PGPR is made from castor oil and is often paired with the emulsifier lecithin, which can be derived from soy, a common allergen. PGPR enhances the functionality of chocolate, as it increases the flow of chocolate into molds and decreases the production of air bubbles in the chocolate. Studies show that PGPR is not carcinogenic, and the Center for Science in the Public Interest has declared it safe for human consumption.

Polysorbate 60: Used as an emulsifier (*see* Emulsifiers), polysorbate 60 comes from corn, palm oil, and petroleum, and is made by a highly complex process. Primarily in animal studies, polysorbate 60 has been shown to harm reproductive health, lead to organ toxicity, and cause cancer in high doses.

Polysorbate 80: An emulsifier used in products such as ice cream to keep ingredients from separating, polysorbate 80 can also be used in creams and lotions intended for personal care. The Environmental Working Group (EWG) reports that this ingredient is linked to cancer as well as nervous system and reproductive toxicity. Furthermore, polysorbate 80 may cause severe nonimmunologic anaphylactoid reactions, with symptoms similar to those of anaphylaxis.

Potassium benzoate and sodium benzoate: *See* Benzoates.

Potassium bisulfate: *See* Sulfites.

Potassium bromate: Banned in almost every country in the world except for the United States and Japan, this additive is used in refined flour to strengthen dough, increasing the volume of bread and rolls. As an oxidizing agent, most of the bromate used breaks down rapidly to form innocuous bromide. If used improperly, however, the residual amount that remains in bread may be harmful if consumed. Bromate causes renal cancer in rats.

Potassium chloride: Often used as a substitute for salt, this chemical compound made of potassium and chlorine is safe, but people with kidney disease or heart disease should consult their doctors about the amount that is safe for them.

Potassium metabisulfite: *See* Sulfites.

Potassium sorbate: *See* Sorbates.

Preservatives: There are three main types of preservatives: antioxidants (such as BHA and BHT), mold inhibitors (such as propionates, found in baked goods and cheese), and sequestrants (such as EDTA, used to prevent changes to the color, odor, and flavor of foods). Food can be preserved naturally with salt, sugar, alcohol, vinegar, and other preservatives.

Propionates (sodium, calcium, and potassium propionate; propionic acid): Propionates are preservatives added to food, such as bread, to inhibit microbial growth. Propionates have been linked to migraines, headaches, and gastrointestinal complaints.

Propyl gallate: An antioxidant preservative used to slow the spoilage of fats and oils. It is often used in combination with BHA and BHT. There is some concern that propyl gallate may cause cancer. Until more studies are done, it's best to avoid products that contain it.

Propylene glycol: This petroleum derivative is used in cosmetics, drugs, and processed foods such as cake mixes, fat-free ice cream and salad dressing. Propylene glycol is an emulsifier, preservative, and humectant (used to retain moisture). The FDA has deemed it safe for consumption. Although it is regarded as having low toxicity in adults, there have been reports regarding toxicity issues in both humans and animals. Propylene glycol may be toxic to the central nervous system, the kidneys, the hematologic (blood) system, and even the heart. It should be avoided by infants. When used topically in products, propylene glycol may irritate the skin. Sensitive individuals and people with eczema should avoid this ingredient.

Propylene glycol monostearate: This cream-colored wax is used as a lubricating agent and emulsifier, a dough conditioner in baked goods, and a stabilizer for essential oils. In animals, it has been shown to produce central nervous system depression and kidney injury in large doses but is considered safe for human consumption (although no long-term studies have been conducted to assess its safety). Allergic reactions have been reported in those with vulvodynia, yeast infections, and interstitial cystitis, and in postmenopausal women using estrogen cream.

Shellac: *See* Confectioners' glaze.

Sodium benzoate: *See* Benzoates.

Sodium bisulfate, sodium metabisulfite: *See* Sulfites.

Sodium caseinate: *See* Casein.

Sodium carboxymethylcellulose: *See* Functional fibers.

Sodium diphosphate: *See* Phosphoric acid, phosphates.

Sodium erythorbate: A food preservative that prevents discoloration, maintains flavor, and reduces the formation of dangerous nitrosamines in foods, particularly in meats, processed meats, and soft drinks. It's considered safe, but sensitive individuals may experience mild side effects, including headaches and flushing.

Sodium hexametaphosphate: Used as an additive to promote stability in ice cream, breakfast cereals, puddings, processed cheese, and even angel food cake. It is also used in the manufacturing of water-softening agents and detergents and can be found in whitening toothpastes.

Sodium nitrite: *See* Nitrates and nitrites.

Sodium pyrophosphate, tetrasodium pyrophosphate: This thickening agent is used in ice cream and instant puddings. According to the Environmental Working Group, studies show that tetrasodium pyrophosphate has been linked to toxicity involving the nervous system.

Sodium sorbate: *See* Sorbates.

Sodium stearoyl lactylate, stearoyl-2-lactylates: This additive is used as a dough strengthener in bread, waffle, and pancake products, and as an emulsifier and stabilizer in icings, fillings, puddings, snack dips, and cheese substitutes. The Center for Science in the Public Interest has deemed sodium stearoyl lactylate as safe.

Sorbates, sorbic acid (potassium, calcium, and sodium sorbate): Sorbates are preservatives found in dairy products and baked products. They are used to prevent the growth of molds, yeasts, and other bacteria. Sorbates have been linked to irritable bowel symptoms, asthma, eczema, and behavior issues in children.

Sorbitan monostearate: This powder is used as an emulsifier in chocolate, ice cream, bread, cake, and coffee. It is considered safe for consumption.

Soy lecithin: Derived from soybeans, this emulsifier is used to improve the texture in a variety of products. Soy is a common genetically modified (GM) food. Because GM foods are a new reality, the long-term health effects have not yet been assessed. Organic soy lecithin is GMO free.

Soybean oil: This oil produced from soybeans is used often in food manufacturing because it seems to have desirable health benefits. It is low in saturated fat, contains no trans fat, and is high in polyunsaturated and monounsaturated fats. The danger in this is that it is highly prone to oxidation and can be damaged easily by heat and light. This oil is often branded as "vegetable oil" and has been refined, blended, and sometimes hydrogenated. It is important to note that unless otherwise stated, soybean oil will be derived from GMO soybeans.

Stevia: This safe noncaloric sweetener is made from the leaves of a Paraguayan herb and is usually found in powder form.

Sucanat: Short for "Sugar Cane Natural," Sucanat is dehydrated sugarcane juice.

Sucralose: Sucralose is another noncaloric sweetener used as a substitute for sugar. Sold as Splenda, it is six hundred times sweeter than table sugar and often recommended to diabetics. It is highly processed, and there have been reports of negative side effects such as gastrointestinal problems and headaches.

Sugar alcohols (erythritol, lactitol, mannitol, sorbitol, and xylitol): Sugar alcohols are used as low-calorie substitutes for sugar and do not promote tooth decay or cause a sudden increase in blood glucose. Sugar alcohols are used mainly to sweeten sugar-free candies, cookies, and chewing gum. Even in small doses, they can aggravate the bowels, causing cramping and diarrhea. They are included in the amount of carbohydrate on the label, either in the total or on a separate line for sugar alcohols.

Erythritol: About 70 percent as sweet as table sugar (sucrose), with almost no calories (0.2 calories per gram). It has a glycemic index score of 0, does not affect blood sugar levels, and does not cause tooth decay or the intestinal upset that other sugar alcohols may cause.

Lactitol: About 40 percent as sweet as sugar, it yields only 2 calories per gram. Lactitol is manufactured from whey, a by-product of cheese making; therefore, individuals who are lactose intolerant should avoid this sugar alcohol.

Mannitol: This prevents chewing gum from absorbing moisture and becoming sticky. It isn't as sweet as sugar and contributes only 2 calories per gram.

Sorbitol: Half as sweet as sugar and often used in chewing gum.

Xylitol: Approved by the FDA in 1963, xylitol occurs naturally in many fruits and vegetables. Produced commercially from plants such as birch and other hardwood trees, it has the same sweetness and bulk as sucrose but with one-third the calories and no unpleasant aftertaste. Xylitol has no known toxic levels, although it may cause diarrhea or mild cramping when too much is consumed.

Xylitol is used in foods such as chewing gum and hard candy, and in oral health products such as throat lozenges, cough syrups, toothpastes, and mouthwashes. Xylitol is poisonous to dogs, so store it properly out of reach.

Sugar, Various Names Used on Food Labels:

- Agave, agave syrup
- Apple juice concentrate
- Barley malt
- Beet juice concentrate
- Brown rice syrup
- Brown sugar
- Cane juice crystals
- Corn syrup
- Crystallized cane juice
- Date sugar
- Dehydrated cane juice crystals
- Demerara sugar
- Dextrose
- Evaporated cane juice
- Evaporated cane juice sugar
- Florida crystals (a trademarked brand)
- Fructose
- Fruit juice concentrate
- Glucose
- Glucose syrup
- High-fructose corn syrup (HFCS)
- High-maltose corn syrup (HMCS)
- Honey
- Invert sugar
- Lactose (milk sugar)
- Malted barley extract
- Maltose
- Milled cane
- Molasses
- Muscovado
- Organic dehydrated cane juice
- Organic oat syrup solids
- Organic palm sugar
- Organic rice syrup
- Organic tapioca syrup
- Palm sugar
- Pure fruit juice concentrate
- Raw cane crystals
- Rice syrup
- Stevia
- Sucanat (a trademarked brand)
- Sucrose
- Sugar
- Tapioca syrup
- Turbinado
- Unbleached crystallized evaporated cane juice
- Unbleached evaporated sugarcane juice crystals
- Unbleached sugarcane
- Unrefined cane juice crystals
- Unsulfured molasses
- Washed cane juice crystals
- Wheat glucose syrup
- White grape juice

Sulfites (sodium sulfite, sulfur dioxide, sodium and potassium bisulfite, sodium and potassium metabisulfite): These can occur naturally in foods or be added to prevent spoilage. Sulfites destroy thiamine (vitamin B_1), and are thought to destroy folic acid, another B vitamin. They have been associated with the full range of food intolerance symptoms, including headaches, irritable bowel symptoms, behavior disturbances, and skin rashes. Sulfites are best known for their effects on asthmatics. Asthmatic individuals can develop bronchospasms after eating foods or drinking wine preserved with sulfur dioxide or other sulfur preservatives.

Tara gum: *See* Gums.

Tartaric acid: *See* Acids.

TBHQ (tertiary butylhydroquinone): A synthetic food-grade antioxidant derived from petroleum, TBHQ is used to increase the shelf life of products and prevent rancidity of fats. TBHQ is used to preserve unsaturated vegetable oils, animal fats, and frozen fish, and is found in some chocolates. It is also used in perfume, varnish, lacquer, and resins. TBHQ has been associated with nausea, vomiting, and tinnitus, and prolonged exposure may cause cancer in lab animals. The FDA limits the amount of TBHQ that can be added to food.

Titanium dioxide (E171): This naturally occurring mineral is used as an artificial color to whiten a wide variety of foods, especially dairy products. It's also used commercially for skin-care products, toothpaste, sunscreen, paper, paint, and more. Allergies to titanium dioxide can range from skin rashes to muscle pain and fatigue.

Trans fat, trans-fatty acids: *See* Partially hydrogenated oil.

Vanillin: The synthetic version of natural vanilla. With vanilla being the most popular flavor in the world and a very labor-intensive (and expensive) ingredient to produce, vanillin quickly became a favored flavoring agent. Most of the vanillin manufactured today is made from petroleum and benzene. The latter, a known carcinogen, goes through a series of chemical refining to produce vanillin.

Yeast extract: *See* Glutamic acid.

Naturally Savvy Approved Brands

Most products are available in Whole Foods, Walmart, Kroger, Safeway, Publix, Fred Meyer, Wegmans, and Stop & Shop stores.

Visit www.naturallysavvy.com for specific stores in your area.

1.2.3 Gluten Free Inc.: www.123glutenfree.com

365 Everyday Value (Whole Foods Brand): www.wholefoodsmarket.com

AH!Laska Chocolate Syrup: www.ahlaska.com

Alden's: www.aldensicecream.com

Alaska's Best: www.alaskasbestsalmonjerky.com

Almond Breeze Almond Milk: www.almondbreeze.com

Almondina: www.almondina.com

Alpsnack-Snack Bars: www.alpsnackinc.com

Alter ECO Fair Trade: www.altereco-usa.com

Alternative Baking: www.alternativebaking.com

Amazing Grass: www.amazinggrass.com

Amy's Kitchen: www.amys.com

Angell Bar: www.angellbar.com

Angie's Kettle Corn: www.angieskettlecorn.com

Annie's: www.annies.com

Arico Natural Foods: www.crisproot.com

Ariel Natural Foods: www.arielfoods.com

Aristo Health: www.aristohealth.com

Arrowhead Mills: www.arrowheadmills.com

Ascenta: www.ascentahealth.com

Attune Foods: www.attunefoods.com

Aunt Gussie's: www.auntgussies.com

Aussie Crunch: www.aussiecrunch.com

Australia's Darrell Lea: www.darrelllea.com

Baby Cakes: www.babycakesnyc.com

Bachman: www.bachmanco.com

Back to Nature: www.backtonaturefoods.com

Baker's: www.kraftbrands.com/bakerschocolate

Balance Bar: www.balance.com

Barbara's: www.barbarasbakery.com

Barleans: www.barleans.com

Bear Fruit Bars: www.morfoods.com

Bear Naked: www.bearnaked.com

Bella's Cookies: www.bellascookies.com

Belly Bar: www.bellybarproducts.com

Ben & Jerry's: www.benjerry.com

Bequet Confections: www.bequetconfections.com

Berkshire Bark: www.berkshirebark.com

Bernod's Spun City: www.bernod.com

Betty Lou's: www.bettylousinc.com

Big Island Organics: www.bigislandorganics.net

Bigelow Tea: www.bigelowtea.com

Bija Bars: www.florahealth.com

Bio-K Plus: www.biokplus.com

Biotta: www.biottajuices.com

Blue Sky: www.blueskysoda.com

Blue Sky Energy: www.blueskyenergyinc.com

Bobo's Oat Bars: www.bobosoatbars.com

Boom Choco Boom: www.enjoylifefoods.com

Bossa Nova: www.bossanovasuperfruits.com

Boston Cookies: www.bostoncookies.com

Bot Beverages: www.botbeverages.com

Boulder Canyon Natural Foods:
www.bouldercanyonfoods.com

Boylan's "The Natural Kind":
www.boylanbottling.com

Bradford Tonic: www.bradfordtonic.com

Brothers: www.brothersallnatural.com

BT Brownies: www.btbaking.com

Bubble Chocolate: www.bubblechocolate.com

Buccaneer: www.gomaxgofoods.com

Buffalo Nickel Wingers:
www.buffalonickelwingers.com

Candy Tree Organic Twists (Whole Foods Market):
www.wholefoods.com

Cape Cod Chips: www.capecodchips.com

Carlson: www.carlsonlabs.com

Carpe Diem: www.carpediem.com

Cascadian Farm: www.cascadianfarm.com

Cheeky Monkey: www.cheekymonkeyorganic.com

Cherrybrook Kitchen:
www.cherrybrookkitchen.com

Chews Better: http://sitekreator.com/kmangold1

Chewy's: www.quakeroats.com

Chocolove: www.chocolove.com

Chris's Cookies: www.chriscookies.com

Chunks O' Fruti: www.nfc-fruti.com

Ciao Bella: www.ciaobellagelato.com

Cindy Klotz Productions:
www.cindyklotzproductions.com

City Girl Country Girl: www.citygirlcountrygirl.net

Clif Bar: www.clifbar.com

Cocoa Cassava: www.cocoacassava.com

Coconut Bliss: www.coconutbliss.com

Cool Cups: www.cool-cups.com

Cool Fruits: www.coolfruits.com

Country Choice Organics:
www.countrychoiceorganic.com

Cracker Jack: www.fritolay.com

Crispy Cat: www.crispycatcandybars.com

Crummy Brothers: www.crummybrothers.com

Dagoba: www.dagobachocolate.com

Dancing Deer Baking Co: www.dancingdeer.com

Das Foods: www.dasfoods.com

Desserts by David Glass: www.davidglass.com

Dirty Chips: www.dirtys.com

Divine Chocolate: www.Divinechocolateusa.com

Divine Treasures: www.dtchocolates.com

Divvies: www.divvies.com

Double Rainbow: www.doublerainbow.com

Dr. Smoothie: www.drsmoothie.com

Dr. Lucy's Cookies: www.drlucys.com

Dr. Oetker Organic: www.oetker.us

Drew's salsa: www.chefdrew.com

Eagle Family Foods: www.eaglebrand.com

Echo Farm Puddings:
www.echofarmpuddings.com

Eco-Planet: www.ecoheavenllc.com/Eco-Planet/
Eco-Planet_Home.html

Embodi: www.drinkembodi.com

Endangered Species: www.chocolatebar.com

Ener-G Foods: www.ener-g.com

Enjoy Life: www.enjoylifefoods.com

Equal Exchange Co-op: www.equalexchange.coop

Erin Baker's Wholesome Baked Goods:
www.bbcookies.com

Essential Living Foods:
www.essentiallivingfoods.com

Ex Drinks: www.exdrinks.com

Fage: www.fageusa.com

FatBoy's Cookie Dough:
www.fatboyscookiedough.com

Fearless Chocolate: www.fearlesschocolate.com

Flamous Brands: www.flamousbrands.com

Flavoroganics: www.flavorganics.com

Flavrz: www.flavrzdrinkmix.com

Florida's Natural: www.ausometreats.com

Food Should Taste Good:
www.foodshouldtastegood.com

Fresh Ginger Ginger Ale by Bruce Cost:
www.freshgingerale.com

Froose: www.froose.com

FrutStix: www.frutstix.com

Frutabu: www.frutabu.com

Funley's: www.funleysdelicious.com

GaGa's: www.gonegaga.net

Garden of Eatin: www.gardenofeatin.com

Genuine Health: www.genuinehealth.com

Gilbert's Goodies:
www.gilbertsgourmetgoodies.com

Glaceau Vitamin Water: www.glaceau.com

Glee Gum: www.gleegum.com

Glenny's: www.glennys.com

Glow: www.glowglutenfree.com

Glutino: www.glutino.com

Go Hunza: www.gohunza.com

Go Naturally: www.hillsidecandy.com

Goldbaum's: www.goldbaums.com

Golden Valley: www.goldenvalleynatural.com

Good Cacao: www.goodcacao.com

Good Health Natural Foods:
www.goodhealthnaturalfoods.com

Good Karma: www.goodkarmafoods.com

Green & Black's: www.greenandblacks.com/us

Grenada Chocolate: www.grenadachocolate.com

Guiltless Gourmet: www.guiltlessgourmet.com

Guittard Chocolate Company: www.guittard.com

Guru: www.guruenergy.com

Gus's Grown-Up Soda: www.drinkgus.com

Haagen-Dazs: www.haagendazs.com

Hank's Gourmet Infusions:
www.hanksbeverages.net

Hansen's Natural: www.hansens.com

Happy Planet: www.happyplanetshots.com

Health Valley: www.healthvalley.com

Healthy Chocolate: www.4noguilt.com

Hero Nutritionals: www.healthyindulgence.com

Himalania: www.himalania.com

Hippie Chips: www.myhippiechips.com

Hodgson Mill: www.hodgsonmill.com

Home Free Organic: www.homefreetreats.com

Honest Tea: www.honesttea.com

Honey Bar: www.honeybar.com

Hubert's Lemonade:
http://www.hubertslemonade.com

Humbles: www.goodhealthnaturalfoods.com

Ian's Natural Foods: www.iansnaturalfoods.com

Immaculate Baking Co.:
www.immaculatebaking.com

Indigo Rabbit: www.indigorabbit.com

Indulge Caramels: www.indulgecaramels.com

International Harvest:
www.internationalharvest.com

IzzeEsque: www.izze.com

Jackie Chan's Tea: www.teatech.com

Jala: www.jalabars.com

Jelly Belly: www.jellybelly.com

Jennie's: www.macaroonking.com

Jokerz: www.gomaxgofoods.com

Jo-Sefs Gluten Free: www.josefsglutenfree.com

Joseph's Lite Cookies:
www.josephslitecookies.com

Julian's Recipe: www.juliansrecipe.com

Julie's Organic: www.juliesorganic.com

Junior Juices: www.drinkjuniorjuice.com

Kashi: www.kashi.com

Katz Gluten Free: www.katzglutenfree.com

Kettle Brand: www.kettlefoods.com

Kid-Fit Chocolate Brownies:
www.kidfitbrownies.com

Kinnikinnick Foods: www.kinnikinnick.com

Kopali Organics: www.kopaliorganics.com

Kozy Shack: www.kozyshack.com

Lake Champlain Chocolates:
www.lakechamplainchocolates.com

LaLoo's Goat milk Ice Cream Company:
www.laloos.com

Larabar: www.larabar.com

Late July Organic Snacks: www.latejuly.com

Laura's Wholesome Junk Food:
www.lauraswholesomejunkfood.com

Lesser Evil: www.lesserevil.com

Let's Do . . . Organic: www.edwardandsons.com

Lily's: www.lilyscakecreations.com

LIV Organic: http://liv-organic.com

Living Fuel Cocochia: www.livingfuel.com

Liz Lovely Cookies: www.lizlovely.com

Loacker: www.loacker.com

Love Candy: www.lovecandy.com

Luna Bars: www.lunabar.com
Lundberg Family: www.lundberg.com
Lydia's Organics: www.lydiasorganics.com
MacaSure: www.macasure.com
MacroLife Naturals: www.macrolifenaturals.com
Madhouse Munchies:
www.madhousemunchies.com
Mahalo: www.gomaxgofoods.com
Mary's Gone Crackers:
www.marysgonecrackers.com
Matt's Cookies: www.mattscookies.net
Mediterranean Snack Foods:
www.mediterraneansnackfoods.com
Michael Seasons: www.seasonssnacks.com
Mi-del: www.midelcookies.com
Mimiccreme: www.mimiccreme.com
Monkey Bars: www.munchythemonkey.com
Moo Chocolate: www.moochocolates.com
Mount Hagen: www.internaturalfoods.com
Mrs. Call's Candy Co.: www.mrscalls.com
Nana's Cookies: www.nanascookiecompany.com
Napoli Boys: www.napoliboys.com
Natural Brew: www.natural-brew.com
Natural Nectar Cookies: www.natural-nectar.com
Natural Vines Licorice:
www.naturalvineslicorice.com
Naturally Nora: www.naturallynora.com
Nature's Choice: www.barbarasbakery.com
Nature's Path Foods: www.naturespath.com
Nature's Select Food Group:
www.natureselectfoodgroup.com

New Morning: www.attunefoods.com
New Sun: www.newsuncookies.com
New Tree: www.newtree.com
Newman's Own Organics:
www.newmansownorganics.com
Nirvana Chocolates: www.nirvanachocolate.com
No Pudge!: www.nopudge.com
Nonuttin': www.nonuttin.com/usa.htm
Nordic Naturals: www.nordicnaturals.com
NuGo: www.nugonutrition.com
Oikos: www.oikosyogurt.com
O.N.E.: www.onedrinks.com
Oogavé: www.oogave.com
Organic Pantry: www.organicpantryshop.com
Organic Prairie: www.organicprairie.com
Organic Valley Co-op: www.organicvalley.com
Original Smart Cookies:
www.originalsmartcookie.com
Oxylent: www.vitalah.com
Pacari Chocolate: www.pacarichocolate.com
Pamela's Products: www.pamelasproducts.com
Panda Licorice: www.pandalicorice.com
Peeled Snacks: www.peeledsnacks.com
Peelu: www.peelu.com
Pirate's Booty: www.piratebrands.com
Pop Chips: www.popchips.com
Pop Corners: www.popcorners.com
Popcorn Indiana: www.popcornindiana.com
Popumz: www.drsearsfamilyessentials.com
Power of Fruit: www.poweroffruit.com
Pretzel Crisps: www.pretzelcrisps.com

Primal Strips: www.primalspiritfoods.com
Purely Decadent: www.turtlemountain.com
Q.Bel: www.Qbelfoods.com
Q-Bees: www.qbtreats.com
R. W. Knudsen: www.knudsenjuice.com
Raw Revolution: http://rawrev.com
Reed's: www.reedsinc.com
Regenie's Organic: www.regenies.com
Rice Dream: www.tastethedream.com
RJ's Licorice: www.rjslicorice.co.nz
Route 11: www.rt11.com
Route 29: www.route29.com
Ruth's Hemp Foods: www.ruthshempfoods.com
Sabrosa Foods Salsa: www.sabrosafoods.com
Sahale Snacks: www.sahalesnacks.com
Salba: www.salba.com
Santa Cruz Organic: www.scojuice.com
Schar: www.schar.com/us
ScharffenBerger: www.Scharffenberger.com
Seeds of Change: www.seedsofchangefoods.com
Seitenbacher: www.seitenbacher.com
Sesmark: www.sesmark.com
Shabtai Gourmet: www.shabtai-gourmet.com
Shaman Chocolates: http://shamangoods.net
ShaSha Co cookies: www.shashabread.com
Sheer Bliss: www.sheerblissicecream.com
Shelton's Beef Jerky: www.sheltons.com
Simply Lemonade: www.simplyorangejuice.com
Simply Organic: http://www.simplyorganic.com
S'Jaaks: www.sjaaks.com

Snikiddy: www.snikiddy.com
Snyder's of Hanover: www.snydersofhanover.com
So Delicious: www.turtlemountain.com
Solea: www.goodhealthnaturalfoods.com
Soyummi: www.soyummifoods.com
St. Claire's: www.stclaires.com
Stacy's: www.stacyssnacks.com
Steaz: www.steaz.com
Stonyfield Organic: www.stonyfield.com
Straus Family Creamery:
    www.strausfamilycreamery.com
Stretch Island Fruit Co: www.stretchislandfruit.com
Sun Cups: www.suncups.com
Sunbutter: www.sunbutter.com
Sunridge Farms: www.sunridgefarms.com
Sunspire: www.sunspire.com
Surf Sweets: www.surfsweets.com
Suzanne's Specialties:
    www.suzannes-specialties.com
Suzie's All Natural Flatbreads:
    www.good-groceries.com
Sweet Earth Chocolates:
    www.sweetearthchocolates.com
Sweet Riot: www.sweetriot.com
Sweet Sam's Baking Co: www.sweetsams.com
Sweet Scoops: www.sweetscoops.com
Tasty Brands: www.tastybaby.com
Tates Cookies: www.tatesbakeshop.com
Teeccino: www.teeccino.com
Tempt Frozen Dessert: www.livingharvest.com

Terra Chips: www.terrachips.com

Terra Nostra Organics:
www.terranostrachocolate.com

The Ginger People: www.gingerpeople.com

Theo chocolate: www.theochocolate.com

Think Thin: www.thinkproducts.com

Three Twins: http://threetwinsicecream.com

TisanoChcolate Tea: www.tisano.com

To Go Brands: www.togobrands.com

Tofutti: www.tofutti.com

Toonie Moonie Organics: www.tooniemoonie.com

Traditional Medicinals: www.tradmed.com

Truly Organic Baking Company:
www.trulyorganicbaking.com

TruSweets: www.trusweets.com

TruWhip: www.truwhip.com

Turkey Hill: www.turkeyhill.com (all natural recipe)

Turtle Mountain: www.turtlemountain.com

Twilight: www.gomaxgofoods.com

Uncle Eddies Cookies:
www.uncleeddiesvegancookies.com

VerMints: www.vermints.com

Vermont Brownie Company:
www.vermontbrowniecompany.com

Vermont Cookie Love:
www.vermontcookielove.com

Vermont Nut Free Chocolates:
www.vermontnutfree.com

Vermont Smoke and Cure:
www.vtsmokeandcure.com

Vintage Plantations: www.vintageplantations.com

Vita Coco: www.vitacoco.com

Vitalicious: www.vitalicious.com

Vitamin Water: www.vitaminwater.com

Walkers: www.walkersus.com

Whole Soy & Co.: www.wholesoyco.com

Wholly Wholesome: www.whollywholesome.com

Wild Harvest: www.wildharvestorganic.com

Woodstock Farms: www.woodstock-farms.com

X-treme Fruit Bites: www.yumyumsnacks.com

Xylichew: www.tundratrading.com

Yoga Chips: www.yogavive.com

Yummy Earth: www.yummyearth.com

Zen Bakery: www.zenbakery.com

Zensoy Organic Soy Pudding: www.zensoy.com

Zevia: www.zevia.com

Zico: www.zico.com

Zola Acai: www.zolaacai.com

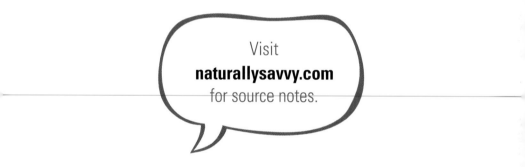

Visit
naturallysavvy.com
for source notes.

Notes

Notes

Notes

Notes

Notes